Type 2 Diabetes cookbook for Beginners

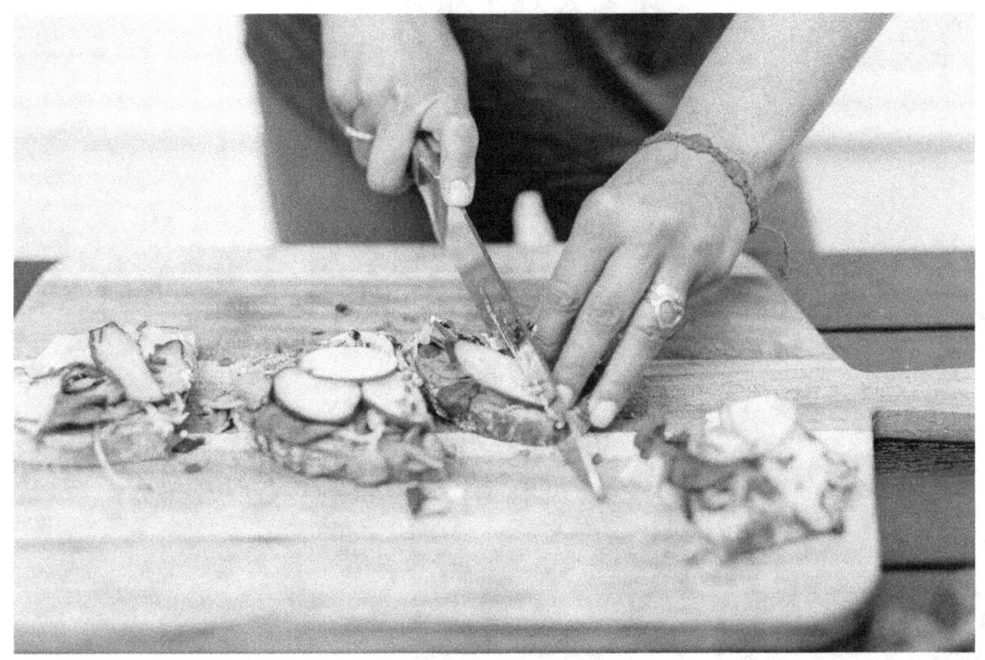

Super Easy Delicious Diabetes Friendly Recipes To Control Blood Sugar Level And Keep it In Check

Caroline Johnson

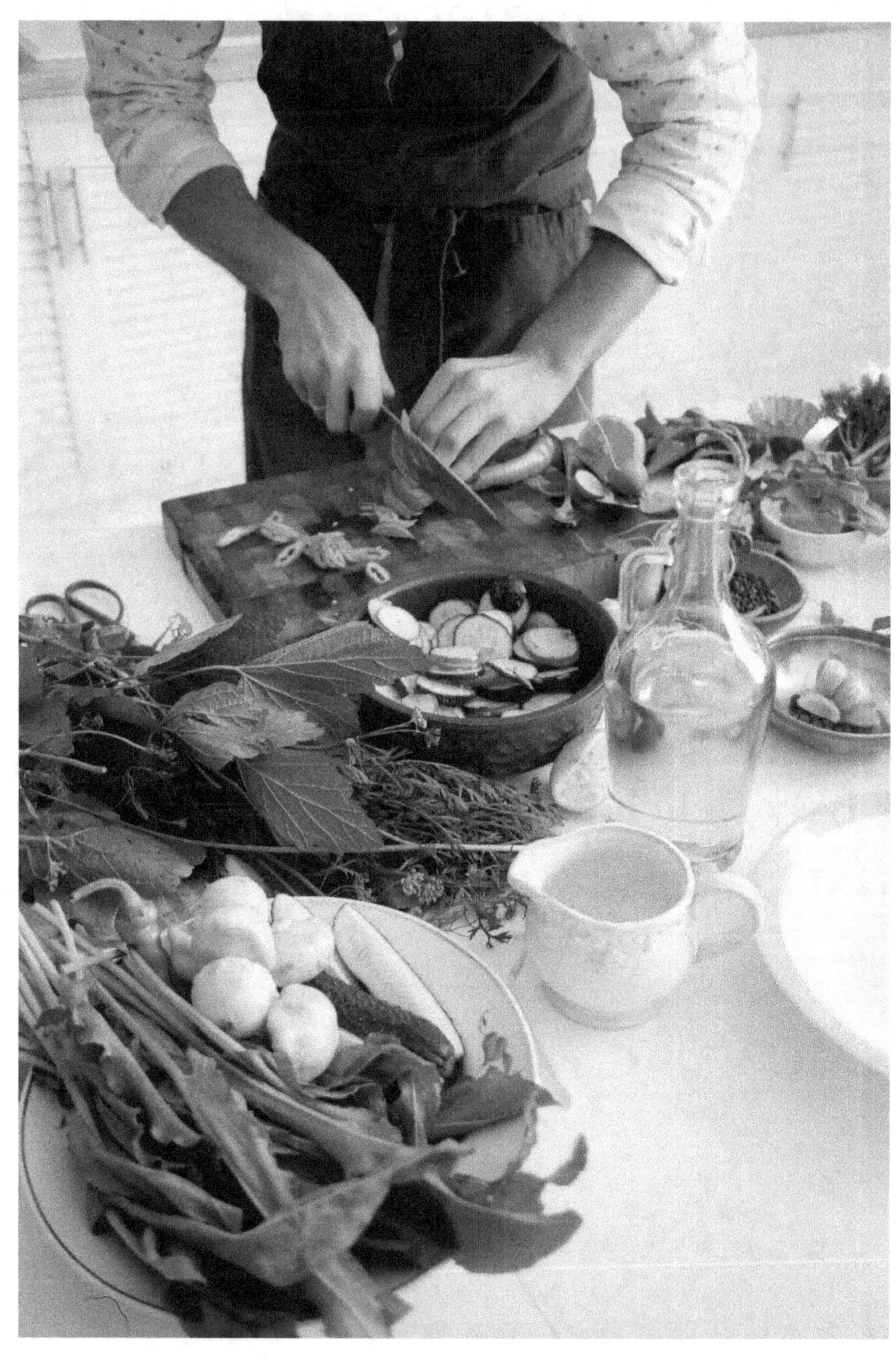

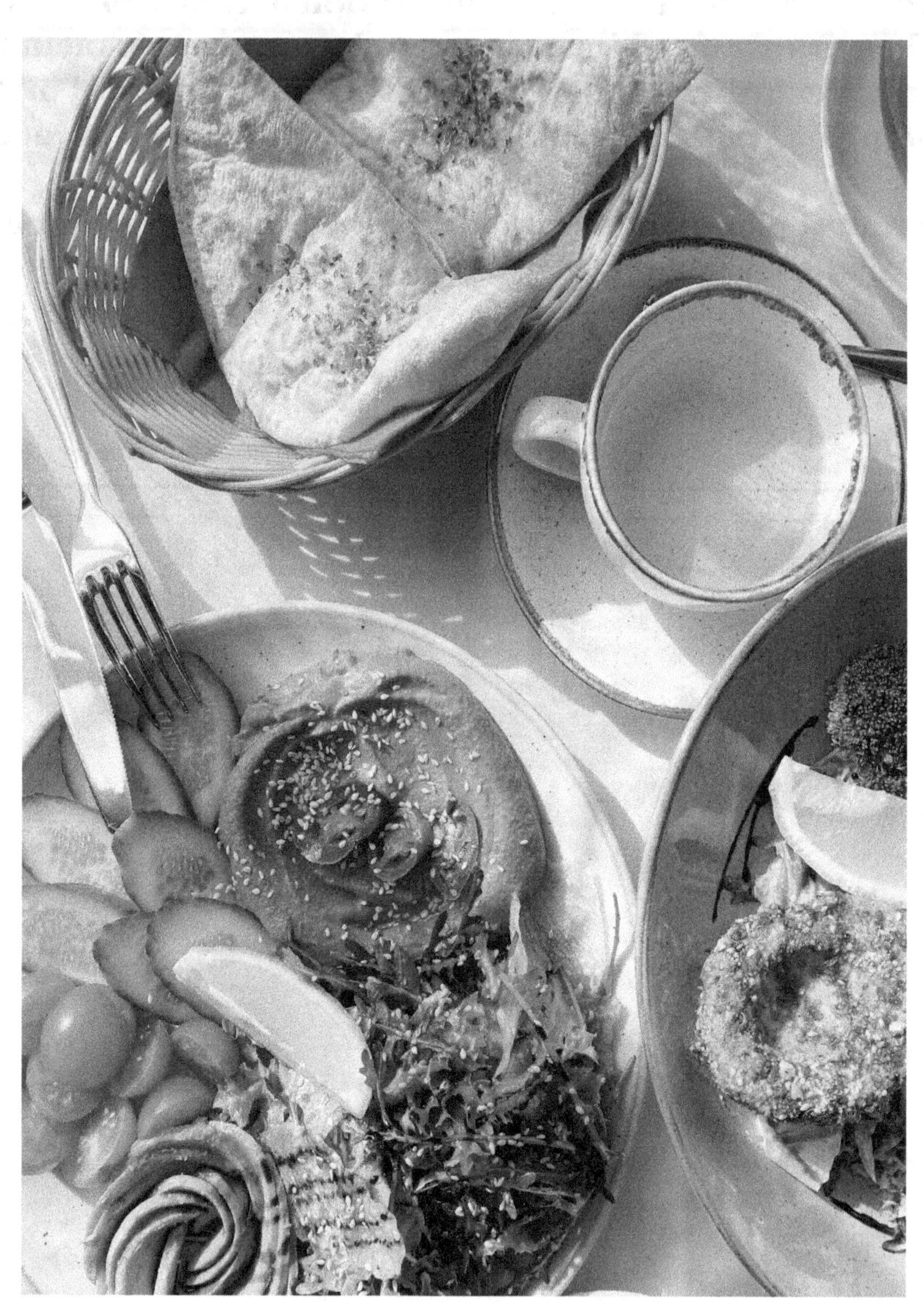

Introduction

Type 2 diabetes affects 537 million people worldwide and it is predicted that by 2030 it will increase to 643 million. As sad as it is, 1 of every 3 persons either have pre or type 2 diabetes. This is a condition where your body lacks the ability to process glucose into energy because your body does not produce insulin or the insulin produced is not functioning.

The news of diabetes is always a shock. You might be going for some random check up and the next thing you are finding out is that you have diabetes. Type 2 diabetes has been the number one cause of kidney failure and lower limb amputation. But you don't have to panic, you can control it by keeping blood sugar level in check and balancing it with the right diet. As tragic as it seems, I need you to believe that it is not a death penalty.

You might be wondering about how to go about your daily diet so you don't complicate things by what you eat. You might be feeling sad that you might no longer have the delicious and tasty food you've been used to. You can have delicious and mouth watering meals and still keep a balanced blood sugar level.

You need not to be worried about how to prepare meals or how to ensure that you have a balanced diet. This book is a product of diverse food research. Research on various foods and their chemical compositions, nutritional value and sugar content has been carried out for you. All you need to do is adhere to these instructions and you will be perfectly fine. You can enjoy great tasty meals and have a happy relationship with food and still have your blood sugar level safe.

This book is a practical guide with pictures to help you understand better when it comes to food preparation. All recipes are carefully explained for better understanding. Go on and satisfy those taste buds in a healthy way. This book also has a special meal plan for you. YOU ARE NOT ALONE IN THIS JOURNEY.

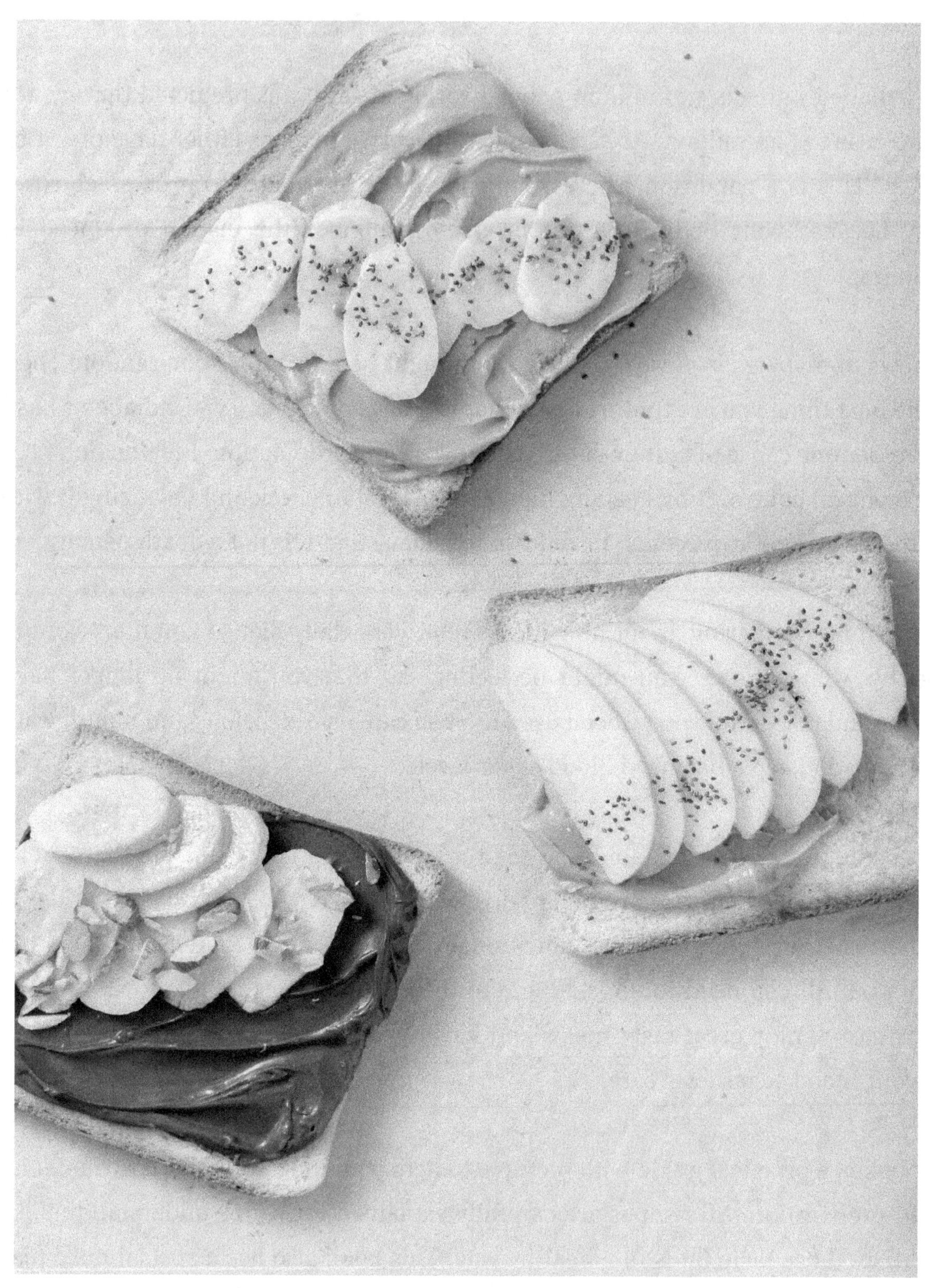

Type 2 diabetes is a chronic metabolic disorder that occurs when the body is unable to produce enough insulin or is unable to use it effectively. Insulin is a hormone produced by the pancreas that helps regulate blood sugar levels by allowing glucose to enter the cells for energy. Without sufficient insulin, glucose accumulates in the bloodstream and can lead to high blood sugar levels, known as hyperglycemia.

There are several factors that contribute to the development of type 2 diabetes, including genetics, lifestyle choices, and obesity. People with a family history of diabetes are at a higher risk of developing the condition. Obesity, especially excess fat around the abdomen, can cause insulin resistance, where the body's cells are less responsive to insulin. This leads to a need for more insulin to maintain normal blood sugar levels, which can eventually exhaust the pancreas and lead to decreased insulin production.

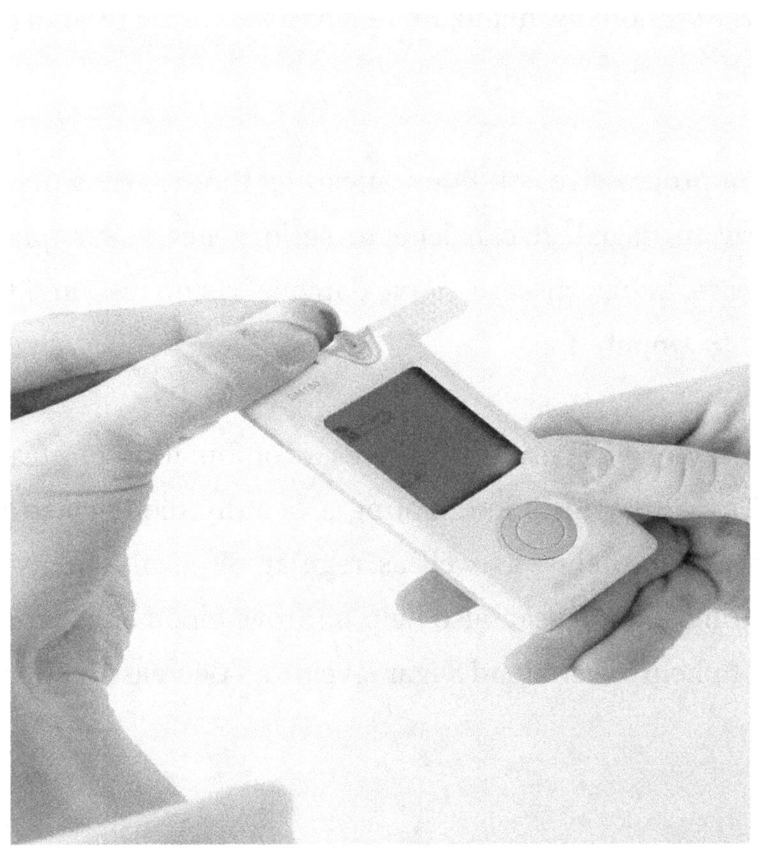

Furthermore, a sedentary lifestyle and a diet high in processed and sugary foods can also increase the risk of developing type 2 diabetes. This is because these factors can contribute to weight gain and insulin resistance.

Symptoms of type 2 diabetes may develop gradually, and some people may not experience any noticeable symptoms at first. However, common symptoms include constant thirst, frequent urination, increased hunger, fatigue, blurred vision, and slow healing of wounds. These symptoms occur because the body is trying to compensate for the lack of insulin by breaking down fat and muscle for energy, leading to weight loss and increased thirst and hunger. High blood sugar levels can also damage blood vessels and nerves, causing numbness and tingling in the hands and feet.

The diagnosis of type 2 diabetes is made through blood tests that measure fasting blood sugar levels. These tests may need to be repeated to confirm the diagnosis as blood sugar levels can fluctuate. Additionally, hemoglobin A1C tests can be used to monitor long-term blood sugar control.

Type 2 diabetes is a progressive condition, meaning that it gets worse over time. If left untreated or poorly managed, it can lead to serious health complications, including cardiovascular disease, kidney disease, nerve damage, vision loss, and foot problems that can ultimately lead to amputation.

Treatment for type 2 diabetes typically involves a combination of lifestyle modifications and medication. These may include adopting a healthy diet rich in fruits, vegetables, whole grains, and lean proteins, as well as regular physical activity. Losing weight if necessary and quitting smoking can also help improve blood sugar control. Medications may be prescribed to help lower blood sugar levels and decrease insulin resistance.

The development of this condition is not sudden and is often a result of a combination of causes and risk factors. Understanding these causes and risk factors is crucial in both preventing and managing type 2 diabetes.

1. Obesity and sedentary lifestyle

Obesity is a major risk factor for type 2 diabetes. It is estimated that about 80% of people with type 2 diabetes are overweight or obese. This is because excess body fat can lead to insulin resistance, which is a key factor in the development of this condition. Additionally, a sedentary lifestyle, which is characterized by lack of physical activity, can also contribute to obesity and increase the risk of type 2 diabetes.

2. Family history and genetics

Family history plays a significant role in the development of type 2 diabetes. Research has shown that if one or both parents have type 2 diabetes, the risk of developing the condition is significantly higher. In addition, certain genetic factors such as the presence of specific gene variants can also increase the risk of developing this disease.

3. Age and ethnicity

Age is another risk factor for type 2 diabetes. As people grow older, their risk of developing type 2 diabetes increases. This is largely due to the natural decline in insulin production and sensitivity that occurs as we age. Additionally, certain ethnic groups, such as African Americans, Asian Americans, and Hispanic Americans, are at a higher risk for type 2 diabetes than other groups.

4. Gestational diabetes

Gestational diabetes is a type of diabetes that develops during pregnancy. Women who have had gestational diabetes are at a higher risk of developing type 2 diabetes later in life. This is because pregnancy can trigger changes in the body that can lead to increased insulin resistance.

5. Unhealthy diet

A diet high in processed foods, saturated fats, and sugar can increase the risk of type 2 diabetes. These unhealthy foods can lead to weight gain and worsen insulin resistance. On the other hand, a diet rich in fruits, vegetables, lean proteins, and whole grains can help prevent and manage type 2 diabetes.

6. Medical conditions

Certain medical conditions can also increase the risk of type 2 diabetes. These include polycystic ovary syndrome (PCOS), sleep apnea, and conditions that affect the pancreas, such as chronic pancreatitis. These conditions can interfere with the body's ability to produce or use insulin, leading to an increased risk of type 2 diabetes.

7. Medications

Some medications, such as corticosteroids and certain antipsychotics, have been linked to an increased risk of type 2 diabetes. This is because these medications may affect insulin production, increase insulin resistance, or cause weight gain.

8. Environmental factors

The environment can also play a role in the development of type 2 diabetes. Exposure to toxins, such as those found in certain chemicals and air pollutants, can impact insulin production and increase the risk of this condition.

In conclusion, type 2 diabetes is a complex condition that can be influenced by a variety of causes and risk factors. While some of these factors, such as age and genetics, cannot be controlled, others, such as obesity and unhealthy lifestyle choices, can be managed to reduce the risk of developing type 2 diabetes. It is important to be aware of these causes and risk factors and make necessary lifestyle changes to prevent or manage this chronic disease.

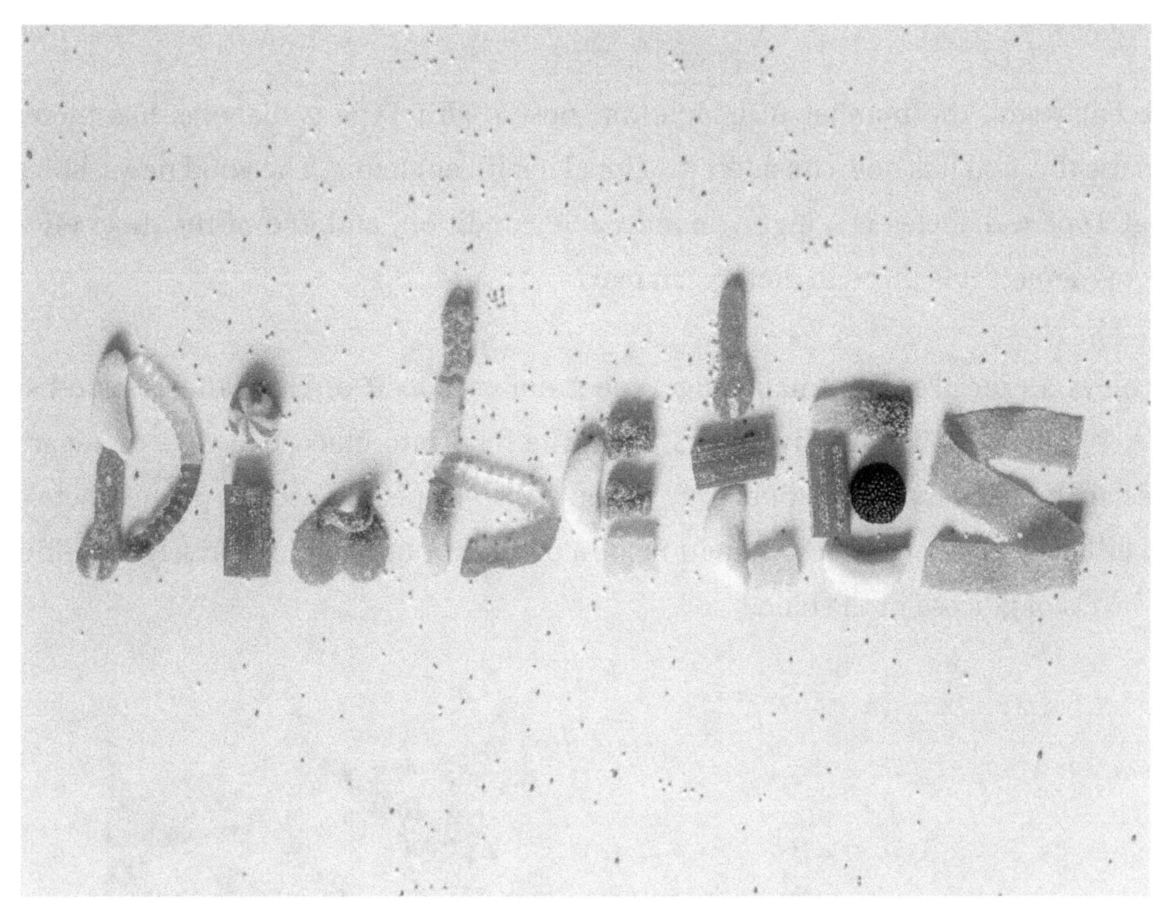

In recent years, the number of people diagnosed with Type 2 diabetes has increased dramatically, and it is now considered a global health epidemic. The good news, however, is that Type 2 diabetes is a highly manageable condition, and one of the most effective ways to manage it is through dietary changes.

Diet plays a crucial role in managing Type 2 diabetes as it directly affects blood sugar levels. When we eat, our body breaks down the food into glucose, a type of sugar that serves as the primary source of energy for our cells. In people with Type 2 diabetes, the body either does not produce enough insulin or cannot utilize it effectively, resulting in high levels of glucose in the blood.

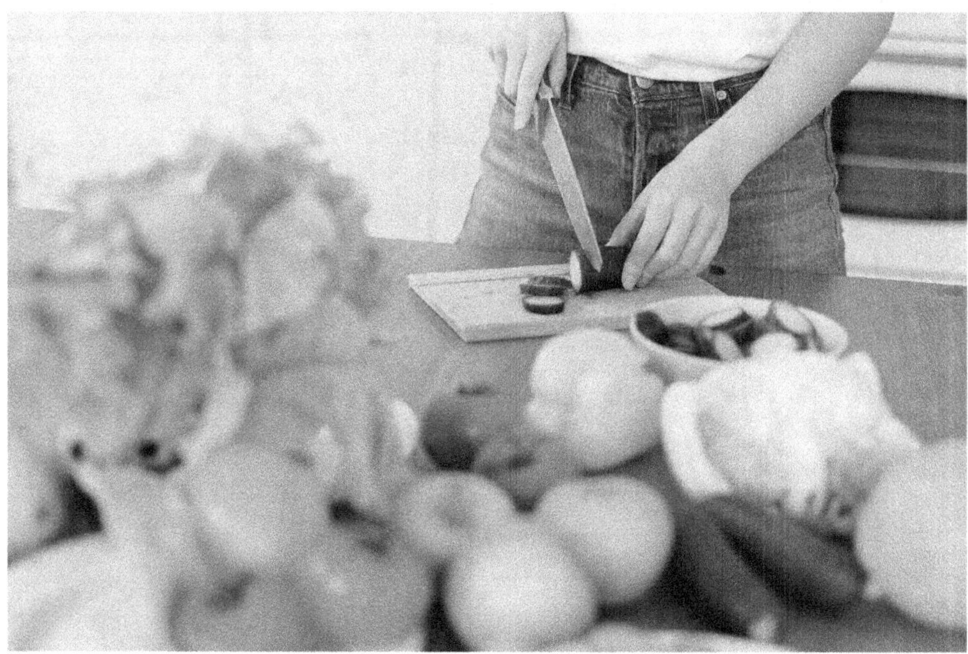

A healthy and balanced diet is essential in managing Type 2 diabetes as it helps control blood sugar levels, maintain a healthy weight, and prevent other health complications associated with the disease. Here are some of the key ways in which diet can play a crucial role in managing Type 2 diabetes:

1. Controlling Carbohydrate Intake:

Carbohydrates have the most significant impact on blood sugar levels, and managing their intake is crucial for people with Type 2 diabetes. Carbohydrates are broken down into glucose during digestion, which raises blood sugar levels. Therefore, a diet high in carbohydrates can lead to sudden spikes in blood sugar levels, making it difficult for people with diabetes to control their condition. Controlling carb intake through portion control, choosing complex carbohydrates like whole grains, fruits, and vegetables, and limiting simple carbs like sugary drinks and processed foods is crucial for managing blood sugar levels.

2. Managing Weight:

Obesity is one of the leading causes of Type 2 diabetes. Eating a healthy and balanced diet can help people with diabetes maintain a healthy weight or lose weight if needed. By choosing nutrient-dense foods such as vegetables, whole grains, and lean proteins, and avoiding calorie-dense and unhealthy foods, one can maintain a healthy weight, which can significantly improve diabetes management.

3. Reducing the Risk of Complications:

Poorly managed Type 2 diabetes can lead to serious health complications, such as heart disease, stroke, nerve damage, and kidney disease. Eating a healthy diet can help reduce the risk of these complications. For instance, a diet rich in heart-healthy foods like fruits, vegetables, and whole grains can help lower the risk of heart disease, which is a common complication of diabetes.

4. Improving Insulin Sensitivity:

Insulin resistance is one of the main causes of Type 2 diabetes. Eating a diet rich in fiber, whole grains, and healthy fats can greatly improve insulin sensitivity, making it easier for the body to utilize the insulin it produces. This, in turn, can help manage blood sugar levels more effectively.

5. Maintaining Overall Health:

A healthy and balanced diet is not only important for managing Type 2 diabetes, but it is also crucial for overall health and well-being. People with diabetes are more prone to other health conditions such as high blood pressure, high cholesterol, and heart disease. A nutritious diet can help manage these conditions and improve overall health, making it easier to manage diabetes.

In summary, diet plays a crucial role in managing Type 2 diabetes. Making healthy dietary choices can greatly improve one's overall health and make it easier to manage diabetes. It is important for people with Type 2 diabetes to work closely with their healthcare providers and registered dietitians to create a personalized meal plan that meets their specific nutritional needs, manages blood sugar levels, and helps to prevent complications. A healthy diet, combined with regular exercise and proper medication, can significantly improve the quality of life for people living with Type 2 diabetes.

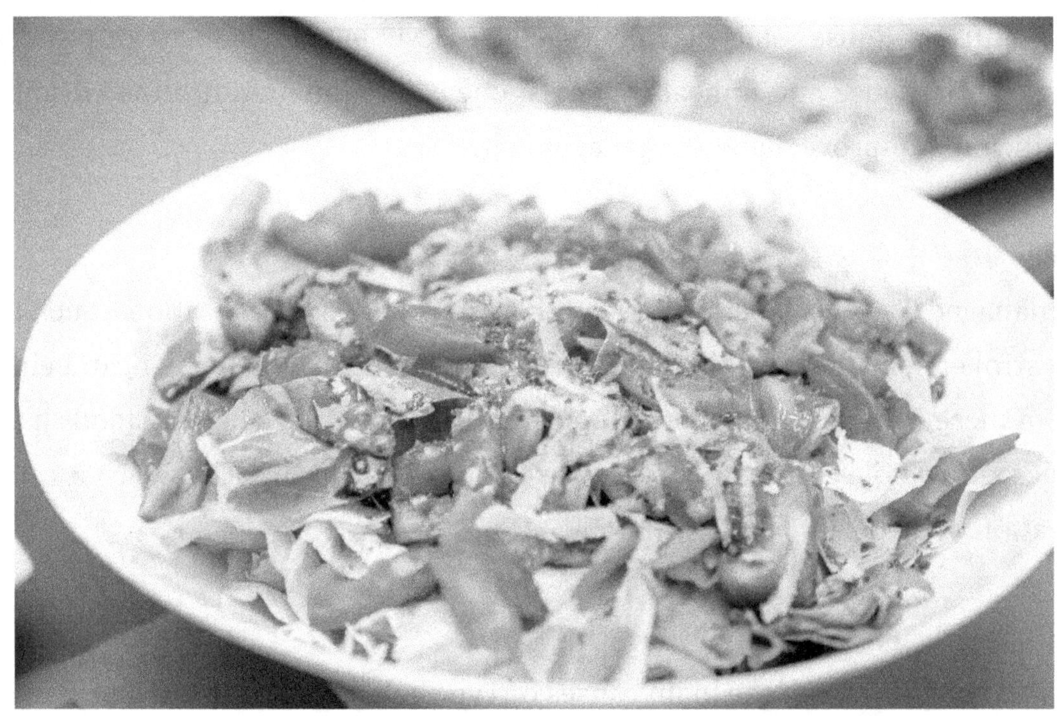

Controlling blood sugar levels is crucial for managing type 2 diabetes and preventing complications such as heart disease, nerve damage, and kidney disease. In this regard, the role of food is paramount as it has a direct impact on blood sugar levels.

Food is the main source of energy for the body, but for people with type 2 diabetes, it is essential to make wise food choices to keep their blood sugar levels stable. The general guide for managing blood sugar levels is to maintain a balanced and healthy diet that includes a variety of nutrient-rich foods such as whole grains, fruits, vegetables, lean proteins, and healthy fats.

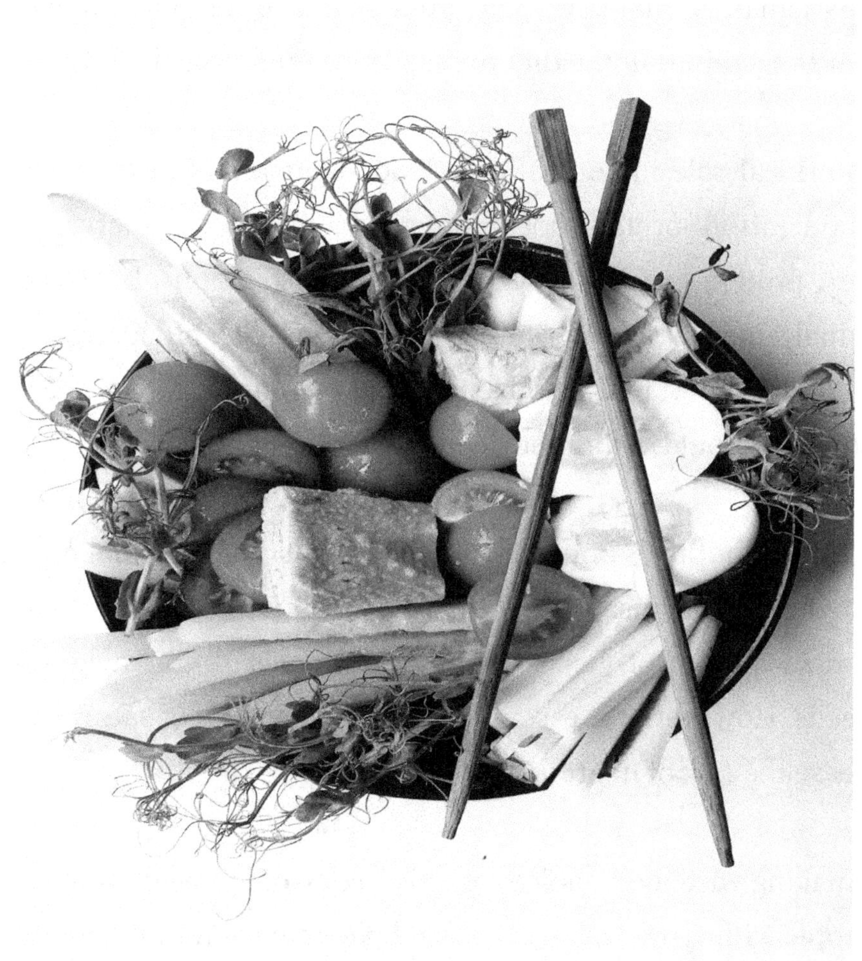

Whole grains are an excellent source of complex carbohydrates that are rich in fiber, vitamins, and minerals. These components help slow down the digestion and absorption of carbohydrates, which leads to a gradual and steady release of glucose into the bloodstream. This helps prevent spikes in blood sugar levels, which is crucial for people with type 2 diabetes. Whole grains such as brown rice, quinoa, and whole-grain bread should replace refined grains like white bread, rice, and pasta in the diet.

Fruits and vegetables are also essential components of a diabetic-friendly diet. These foods are low in calories and rich in fiber, antioxidants, and other essential nutrients. They have a low glycemic index, which means they do not cause a sharp increase in blood sugar levels. However, it is essential to limit the intake of fruits and vegetables with a high sugar content, such as bananas, mangoes, and potatoes. The key is to include a variety of colorful fruits and vegetables in the diet to reap their numerous health benefits.

Protein plays a critical role in controlling blood sugar levels in type 2 diabetes. When consumed in moderation, protein does not cause a significant increase in blood sugar levels. Moreover, protein can help slow down the absorption of carbohydrates, which leads to a gradual and steady release of glucose into the bloodstream. Lean protein sources such as fish, poultry, tofu, and legumes are recommended, while high-fat protein sources like red meat should be limited.

Healthy fats are another important component of a diabetic-friendly diet. Monounsaturated and polyunsaturated fats have numerous health benefits, including improving blood sugar control. Foods rich in these types of fats include avocados, olive oil, nuts, and seeds. However, it is essential to limit the intake of saturated and trans fats, which can increase the risk of heart disease.

In addition to making wise food choices, portion control is essential for managing blood sugar levels. People with type 2 diabetes should pay attention to the amount of food they consume at each meal and aim to eat smaller, more frequent meals throughout the day. This helps prevent large spikes in blood sugar levels that can occur when eating large meals.

Lastly, it is also essential to pay attention to the timing of meals and snacks. Consistency is key when it comes to managing blood sugar levels in type 2 diabetes. Eating meals and snacks at regular intervals and not skipping meals can help keep blood sugar levels stable.

Food plays a crucial role in controlling blood sugar levels in type 2 diabetes. Following a balanced and healthy diet that includes whole grains, fruits, vegetables, lean proteins, and healthy fats is essential for managing this chronic condition. Additionally, portion control and consistent meal timings are equally important. By making sensible food choices and adopting healthy eating habits, people with type 2 diabetes can effectively manage their blood sugar levels and lead a healthier

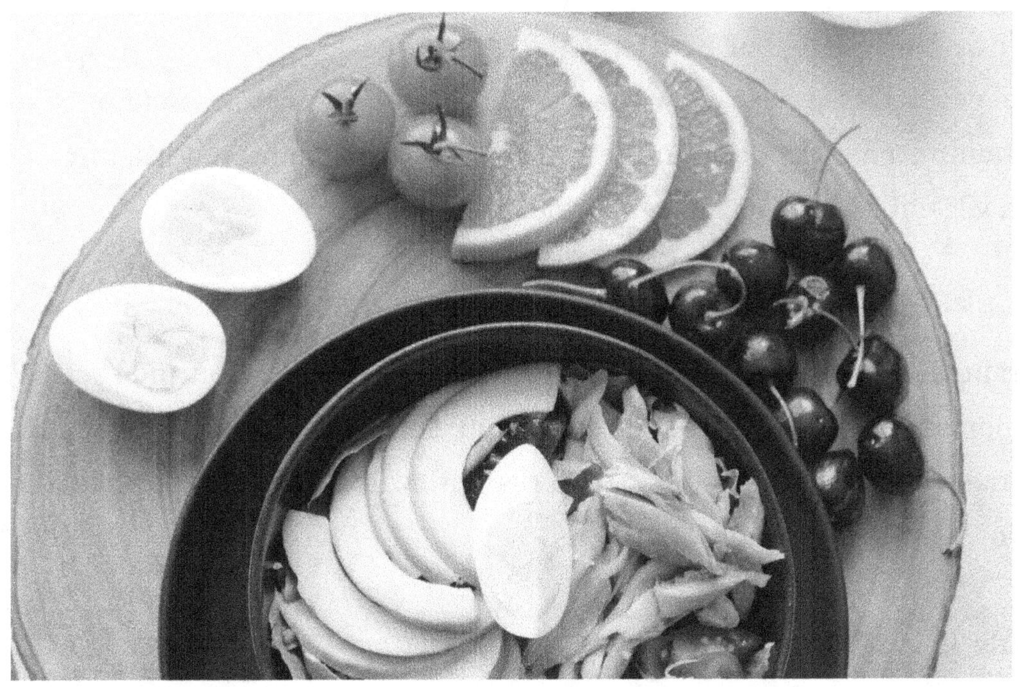

Tips for Maintaining a Well-Balanced Diet

Maintaining a well-balanced diet is essential for overall health and well-being. A balanced diet provides the body with the necessary nutrients, vitamins, and minerals to function at its best. It also helps with weight management, energy levels, and disease prevention. Here are some tips for maintaining a well-balanced diet:

1. Eat a Variety of Foods

The key to a balanced diet is variety. Consuming a variety of foods ensures that your body gets all the necessary nutrients it needs. Include different types of fruits, vegetables, whole grains, lean protein sources, and healthy fats in your meals. Try new foods and experiment with different recipes to keep your meals interesting.

2. Get Your Daily Dose of Fruits and Vegetables

Fruits and vegetables are packed with essential vitamins, minerals, and fiber that are vital for maintaining a healthy body and preventing diseases. Aim for at least five servings of fruits and vegetables each day to get a wide range of nutrients.

3. Choose Whole Grains

Whole grains are an excellent source of fiber, which aids in digestion and keeps you feeling fuller for longer. They also provide essential nutrients, such as iron and B vitamins. Swap refined grains like white bread, pasta, and rice with whole grain options like whole-wheat bread, brown rice, and quinoa.

4. Include Lean Protein Sources

Protein is crucial for building and repairing tissues in the body, as well as for maintaining a healthy immune system. Choose lean protein sources like fish, chicken, turkey, beans, legumes, and tofu. Limit your intake of red and processed meats, which have been linked to an increased risk of heart disease and other health problems.

5. Don't Forget Healthy Fats

Although it's often associated with unhealthy foods, fat is an essential part of a balanced diet. Healthy fats like avocados, nuts, and olive oil provide the body with essential fatty acids, which help protect the heart and maintain brain health. However, it's essential to limit your intake of saturated and trans fats, which can negatively impact heart health.

6. Moderation is Key

Maintaining a balanced diet is not about strict rules or deprivation. It's about moderation and making mindful choices. It's okay to indulge in your favorite foods occasionally, but try to limit your portions and balance it out with healthier options throughout the day.

7. Drink Plenty of Water

Staying hydrated is essential for a healthy body. Drinking enough water helps boost metabolism, aids digestion, and keeps the body functioning properly. Aim for at least eight glasses of water per day and limit sugary drinks like sodas and juices.

8. Limit Processed and Fast Foods

Processed and fast foods are often high in unhealthy fats, added sugars, and sodium. These foods provide little to no nutritional value and can contribute to weight gain and chronic health conditions. Instead, opt for whole, unprocessed foods whenever possible.

9. Plan and Prepare Meals Ahead of Time

Meal planning and preparation can help you make healthier choices and save time and money. Plan your meals for the week, make a grocery list, and prep ingredients in advance. This will make it easier to stick to a balanced diet and avoid relying on quick, unhealthy options when you're short on time.

10. Listen to Your Body

Everyone's dietary needs and preferences are different. It's essential to listen to your body and make adjustments to your diet as needed. If you have any food allergies, intolerances, or specific dietary restrictions, make sure to find suitable alternatives and consult a healthcare professional for advice on how to maintain a balanced diet.

Processed and high-sugar foods have become a staple in our modern diet due to their convenience and availability. However, these types of foods have been linked to numerous health issues, including obesity, type 2 diabetes, and heart disease. As a result, many people are looking for healthier and more natural alternatives to processed and high-sugar foods. Here are some options to consider:

1. Whole Foods: Instead of processed foods that have gone through multiple stages of refinement, opt for whole foods that are in their natural state. This includes fruits, vegetables, whole grains, and lean proteins. These foods contain essential nutrients, fiber, and antioxidants that are vital for maintaining good health.

2. Homemade Meals: Making meals from scratch using fresh, whole ingredients is a great way to avoid processed foods. It allows you to control the ingredients and portion sizes, cutting down on added sugars and unhealthy additives. You can experiment with different recipes and flavors, making your meals more enjoyable and nutritious.

3. Natural Sweeteners: Instead of using refined sugars, consider using natural sweeteners like honey, maple syrup, or dates in your meals and desserts. These options contain more nutrients and have a lower glycemic index, which means they won't cause a spike in blood sugar levels.

4. Snack on Fruits and Nuts: Most processed snacks are high in sugar and unhealthy fats. Instead, try snacking on fresh fruits and nuts, which are packed with nutrients and healthy fats. They are also easy to pack and carry around for a mid-day energy boost.

5. Alternative to Processed Meats: Processed meats, such as bacon, sausages, and deli meats, are highly processed and often contain added sugars and unhealthy preservatives. Replace these with lean proteins like chicken, fish, and tofu, which are unprocessed and a healthier option.

6. Choose Whole-Grain Products: Instead of refined grains like white bread and pasta, opt for whole-grain alternatives such as brown rice, whole-wheat bread, and quinoa. These options contain more fiber, vitamins, and minerals, making them a healthier choice.

7. Swap Soda for Infused Water: Sodas and other sugary drinks are a significant source of added sugars in the diet. Replace these with infused water, which adds natural flavors without any added sugars or artificial sweeteners.

8. Make Your Own Condiments and Sauces: Many condiments and sauces, such as ketchup, barbecue sauce, and salad dressings, are loaded with sugar and unhealthy additives. Making them at home using fresh ingredients allows you to control the sugar and add healthier options like herbs, spices, and olive oil.

9. Try Fermented Foods: Fermented foods like yogurt, kefir, and sauerkraut contain probiotics, which are beneficial for gut health. These options provide a healthier alternative to processed dairy products, which can be high in added sugars.

10. Satisfy Your Sweet Tooth with Fruits: Instead of reaching for processed sweets like cookies and candies, satisfy your sweet tooth with fruits like berries, apples, and bananas. These provide natural sweetness and are also rich in nutrients and antioxidants.

As a person living with type 2 diabetes, it is essential to understand that what you eat plays a crucial role in managing your condition. Maintaining a healthy and balanced diet is key to controlling your blood sugar levels, reducing the risk of diabetes-related complications, and improving overall health. A well-planned diabetes-friendly diet should focus on specific nutrients that are essential for managing diabetes effectively. In this article, we will discuss the basics of a diabetes-friendly diet and the nutrients that you should focus on to improve your overall well-being.

1. Carbohydrates:

Carbohydrates are the body's main source of energy, and they have the most significant impact on blood sugar levels. Therefore, it is crucial to choose the right types and amounts of carbohydrates. Complex carbohydrates such as whole grains, fruits, vegetables, and legumes are better choices as they are digested more slowly and have a lesser impact on blood sugar levels. On the other hand, simple carbohydrates such as sweets, sugary drinks, and processed foods should be limited as they can cause a sharp rise in blood sugar levels.

2. Fiber:

Fiber is an essential nutrient for people with diabetes as it helps in managing blood sugar levels, reduces the risk of heart disease, and aids in weight management. It also helps in controlling hunger and promotes a feeling of fullness. Foods high in fiber include whole grains, fruits, vegetables, nuts, seeds, and legumes. Aim to incorporate at least 25-30 grams of fiber in your daily diet.

3. Protein:

Protein plays a vital role in building and repairing tissues, maintaining muscle mass, and keeping you feeling full. When it comes to diabetes, protein can help slow down the absorption of carbohydrates, which in turn helps in managing blood sugar levels. Good sources of protein for a diabetes-friendly diet include lean meats, poultry, fish, eggs, tofu, and low-fat dairy products. It is recommended to include a serving of protein with each meal.

4. Healthy Fats:

Contrary to popular belief, not all fats are bad. Healthy fats such as monounsaturated and polyunsaturated fats have numerous health benefits, including lowering bad cholesterol levels, improving heart health, and stabilizing blood sugar levels. Foods high in healthy fats include avocados, olive oil, nuts, seeds, fatty fish, and tofu. However, it is crucial to keep portion sizes in check as fats are high in calories.

5. Vitamins and minerals:

Vitamins and minerals are essential for overall health, and they play a crucial role in managing diabetes. Some key nutrients to focus on include:

- Vitamin D: Helps in maintaining healthy bones and may help improve insulin sensitivity. Good sources include fatty fish, egg yolks, and fortified foods.
- Magnesium: Helps in regulating blood sugar levels and can be found in dark leafy greens, nuts, seeds, and whole grains.
- Potassium: Aids in controlling blood pressure and can be found in fruits, vegetables, and dairy products.
- Calcium: Helps in maintaining bone health and can be found in dairy products, green leafy vegetables, and fortified foods.

It is important to include a variety of fruits, vegetables, whole grains, lean protein, and healthy fats to ensure you are getting a good mix of vitamins and minerals in your diet.

In addition to focusing on these nutrients, it is equally important for people with diabetes to monitor their portion sizes, limit added sugars and sodium, and stay hydrated by drinking plenty of water. Consulting a registered dietitian can also be beneficial in creating a personalized diabetes-friendly meal plan.

A well-balanced and nutritious diet is crucial for managing type 2 diabetes effectively. By focusing on the right nutrients, you can maintain stable blood sugar levels, reduce the risk of complications, and lead a healthy and fulfilling lifestyle. Remember to make small, sustainable changes to your diet, and consult your healthcare team for guidance on managing your diabetes through proper nutrition.

Type 2 diabetes is a chronic condition in which the body's ability to produce and use insulin, the hormone responsible for regulating blood sugar levels, is impaired. It is important for individuals with type 2 diabetes to carefully monitor their diet, as certain foods can have a major impact on blood sugar levels. In order to properly manage the disease, it is crucial to limit or avoid certain foods that can worsen the condition.

1. Processed and refined carbohydrates: Foods such as white bread, pasta, rice, and sugary cereals are high in carbohydrates and have a high glycemic index, meaning they cause a rapid spike in blood sugar levels. This can make it difficult for the body to regulate blood sugar and insulin levels. Instead, opt for whole grain and complex carbohydrate sources such as oatmeal, quinoa, and brown rice.

2. Sugar-sweetened beverages: Regular consumption of sugary drinks like soda, fruit juices, and sports drinks can significantly increase the risk of developing type 2 diabetes. These beverages are loaded with added sugar and lack any nutritional value. Water is the best choice for staying hydrated, or try adding fresh fruit slices or herbs for flavor.

3. Fried and fatty foods: Foods high in saturated and trans fats, such as fried foods, burgers, and fatty red meats, can contribute to insulin resistance and increase the risk of heart disease. Instead, opt for lean proteins like chicken, fish, and tofu, and choose heart-healthy fats such as avocados, olive oil, and nuts.

4. Processed and high-sodium foods: Processed foods like deli meats, canned soups, and frozen meals are often high in sodium, which can lead to high blood pressure and increase the risk of heart disease. These foods are also typically lacking in essential nutrients and may contain added sugars and unhealthy fats. It is best to choose fresh, whole foods and limit processed options.

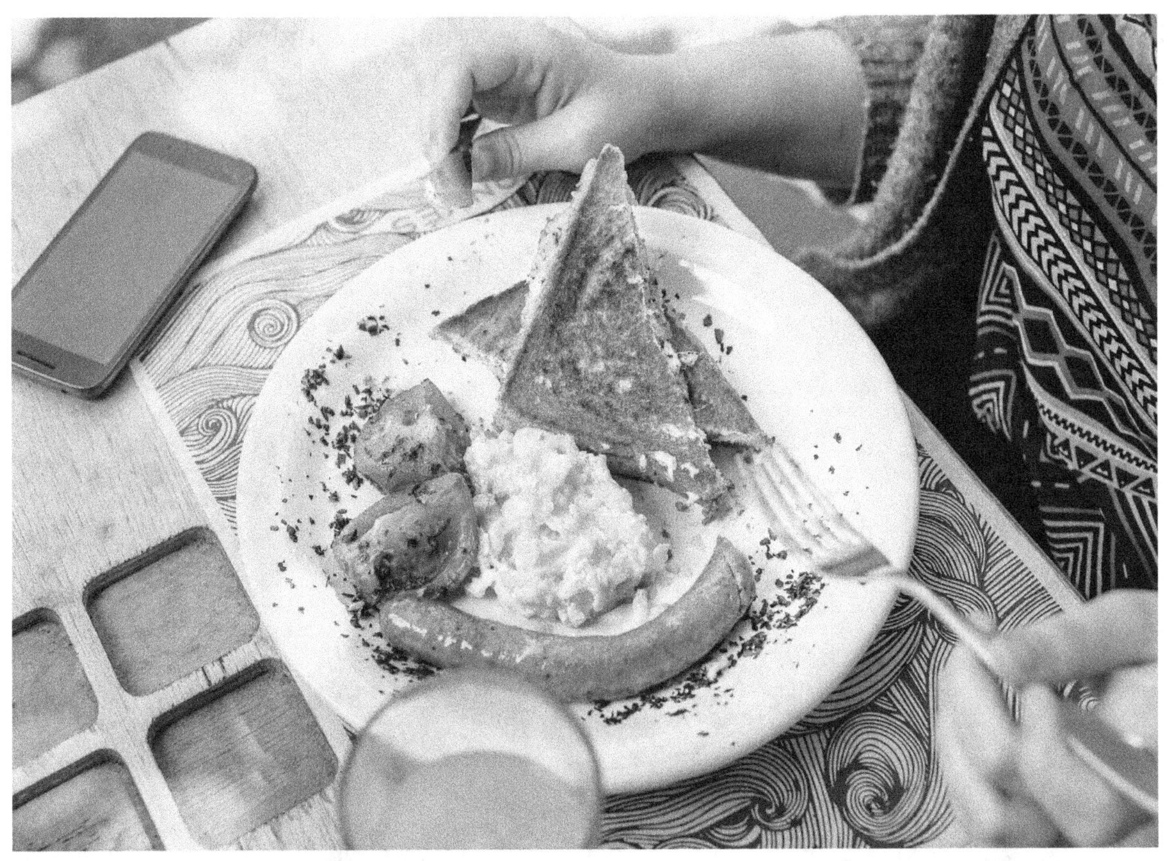

5. Alcohol: Moderate alcohol consumption may have some health benefits, but excessive consumption can lead to an increase in blood sugar levels and can also interfere with diabetes medication. It is important for individuals with type 2 diabetes to limit their alcohol intake and monitor blood sugar levels when consuming alcoholic beverages.

In addition to limiting or avoiding these specific foods, it is important for individuals with type 2 diabetes to maintain a well-balanced diet that includes plenty of fruits, vegetables, whole grains, and lean proteins. It is also important to control portion sizes and monitor carbohydrate intake, as carbohydrates have the biggest impact on blood sugar levels.

Individuals with type 2 diabetes should limit or avoid processed and refined carbohydrates, sugar-sweetened beverages, fried and fatty foods, processed and high-sodium foods, and excessive alcohol consumption. Instead, they should focus on incorporating whole, nutritious foods into their diet and monitoring their blood sugar levels to effectively manage their condition. Consultation with a registered dietitian or certified diabetes educator can also provide personalized guidance and support in creating a healthy and diabetes-friendly meal plan.

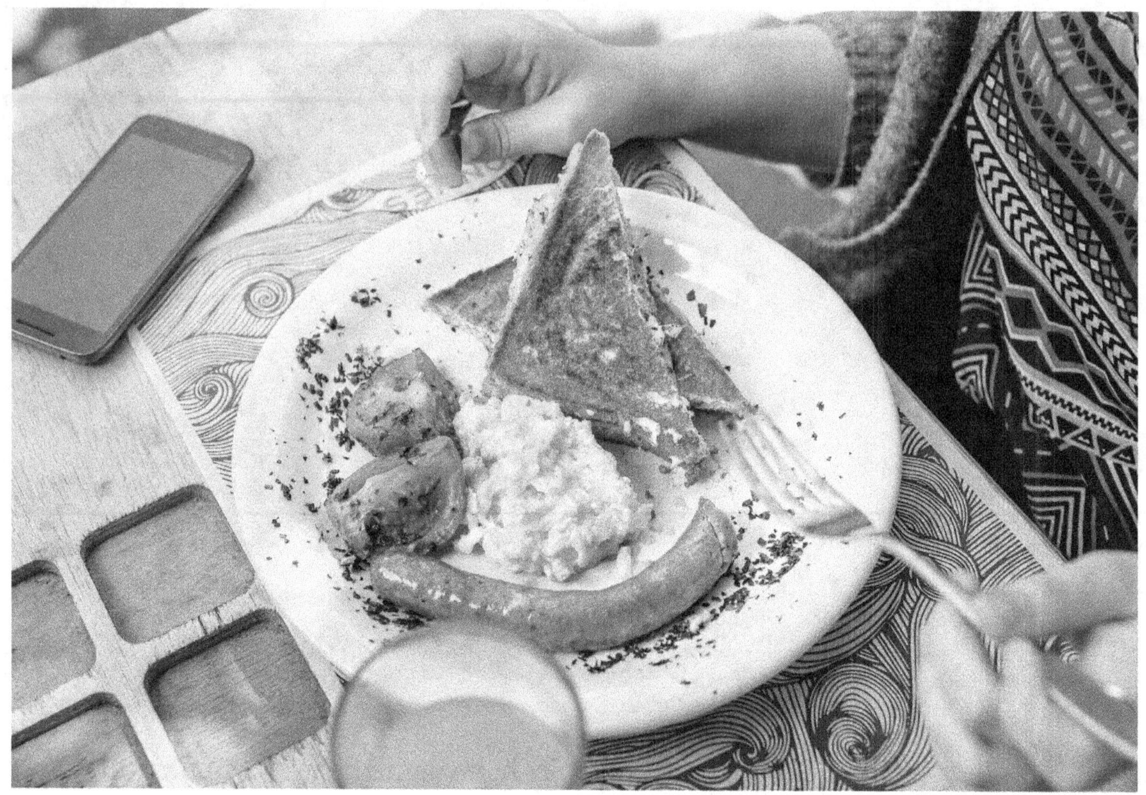

As a type 2 diabetes patient, it is essential for you to manage your diet in order to maintain stable blood sugar levels and prevent any future complications. One of the key components of a healthy diet for diabetes is cutting down on saturated and trans fats. These types of fats have been linked to an increased risk of heart disease and can worsen your diabetes symptoms.

Saturated fats are primarily found in animal products such as red meat, full-fat dairy, and butter. Trans fats, on the other hand, are mainly found in processed foods such as fried foods, baked goods, and packaged snacks. These fats raise your cholesterol levels and may also increase inflammation in the body, which can lead to insulin resistance.

Here are some tips to help you effectively cut down on saturated and trans fats in your diet:

1. Choose lean protein sources: When it comes to selecting your protein sources, opt for lean options such as chicken, turkey, fish, and plant-based options like beans, lentils, and tofu. These are lower in saturated fats compared to red meat and processed meats like bacon and sausage.

2. Switch to low-fat or fat-free dairy: Full-fat dairy products are high in saturated fats, which can negatively impact your cholesterol levels. Make a switch to low-fat or fat-free dairy options such as skim milk, low-fat yogurt, and reduced-fat cheese.

3. Use healthy cooking methods: Avoid cooking your food in unhealthy sources of fat such as butter or lard. Instead, use healthier options like olive oil, canola oil, or avocado oil. These oils are higher in unsaturated fats, which are considered healthier for the heart.

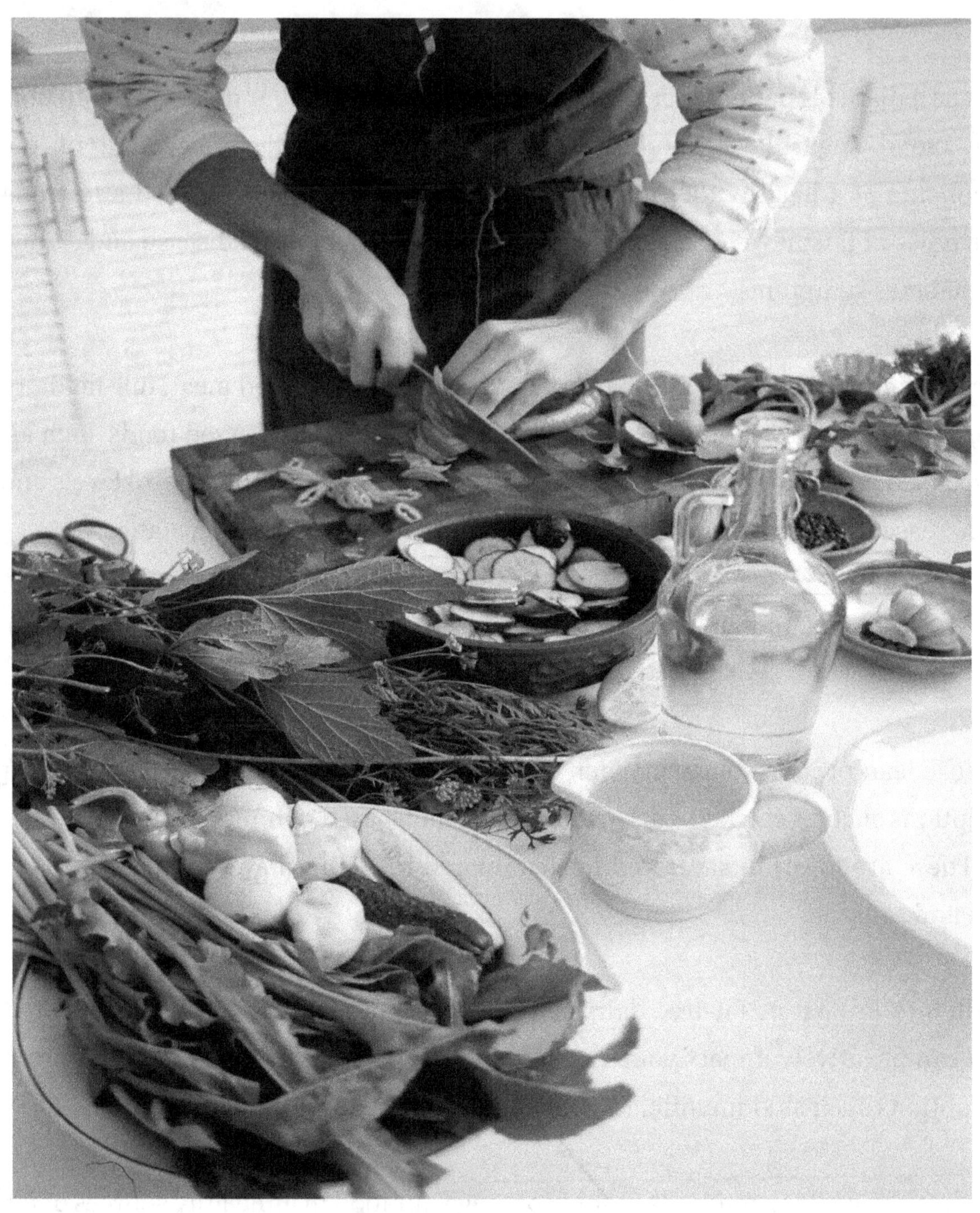

4. Read labels carefully: When purchasing packaged foods, it is important to read the labels carefully. Look for foods that are labeled as "trans-fat-free" or have 0 grams of trans fat per serving. However, keep in mind that even if a food is labeled as "trans-fat-free," it may still contain small amounts of trans fat.

5. Fill up on fruits and vegetables: Fruits and vegetables are naturally low in saturated and trans fats, making them an excellent choice for diabetes patients. Aim to fill half of your plate with a variety of colorful fruits and vegetables to increase your intake of vitamins, minerals, and antioxidants.

6. Make homemade meals: Cooking your meals at home gives you more control over the ingredients and can help you avoid unhealthy fats. Experiment with different herbs and spices to add flavor to your meals instead of relying on high-fat ingredients.

In addition to cutting down on saturated and trans fats, it is also important to maintain a balanced diet with a variety of whole grains, lean protein, and healthy fats. Regular physical activity also plays a crucial role in managing type 2 diabetes.

I hope these tips will help you make healthier choices and manage your diabetes effectively. Remember to also consult with your doctor or a registered dietitian for personalized dietary advice.

Visit Caroline Johnson Author Central page for more health books

Part 3: Breakfast Recipes

Leafy Green and Avocado Omelet

Leafy Green and Avocado Omelet Recipe:

Ingredients:

- 2 large eggs
- 1/4 cup chopped leafy greens (such as spinach, kale, or Swiss chard)
- 1/4 avocado, diced
- 1/4 cup diced tomatoes
- 1/4 cup shredded cheddar cheese
- 1 tbsp olive oil
- Salt and pepper to taste

Instructions:

1. In a small bowl, beat 2 eggs until they are fluffy and well combined.

2. In a separate bowl, mix together the chopped leafy greens, diced avocado, diced tomatoes, and shredded cheddar cheese.

3. Heat 1 tbsp of olive oil in a nonstick skillet over medium-high heat.

4. Pour the beaten eggs into the skillet and swirl to make a thin even layer.

5. Let the eggs cook for about a minute or until the bottom is golden brown.

6. Gently flip the omelet over to cook the other side for another minute.

7. Once the omelet is cooked through, add the leafy green and avocado mixture on one side of the omelet.

8. Season with salt and pepper to taste.

9. Using a spatula, fold the other half of the omelet over the mixture to create a half-moon shape.

10. Let the omelet cook for an additional minute or until the cheese is melted.

11. Carefully slide the omelet onto a plate and let it cool for a minute before serving.

This leafy green and avocado omelet is a delicious and nutritious option for a diabetes-friendly breakfast. The leafy greens provide fiber and essential vitamins, while the avocado adds healthy fats and creaminess. The combination of protein and healthy fats makes this omelet a great option for stabilizing blood sugar levels. Enjoy with a side of whole grain toast or fresh fruit for a satisfying and balanced meal.

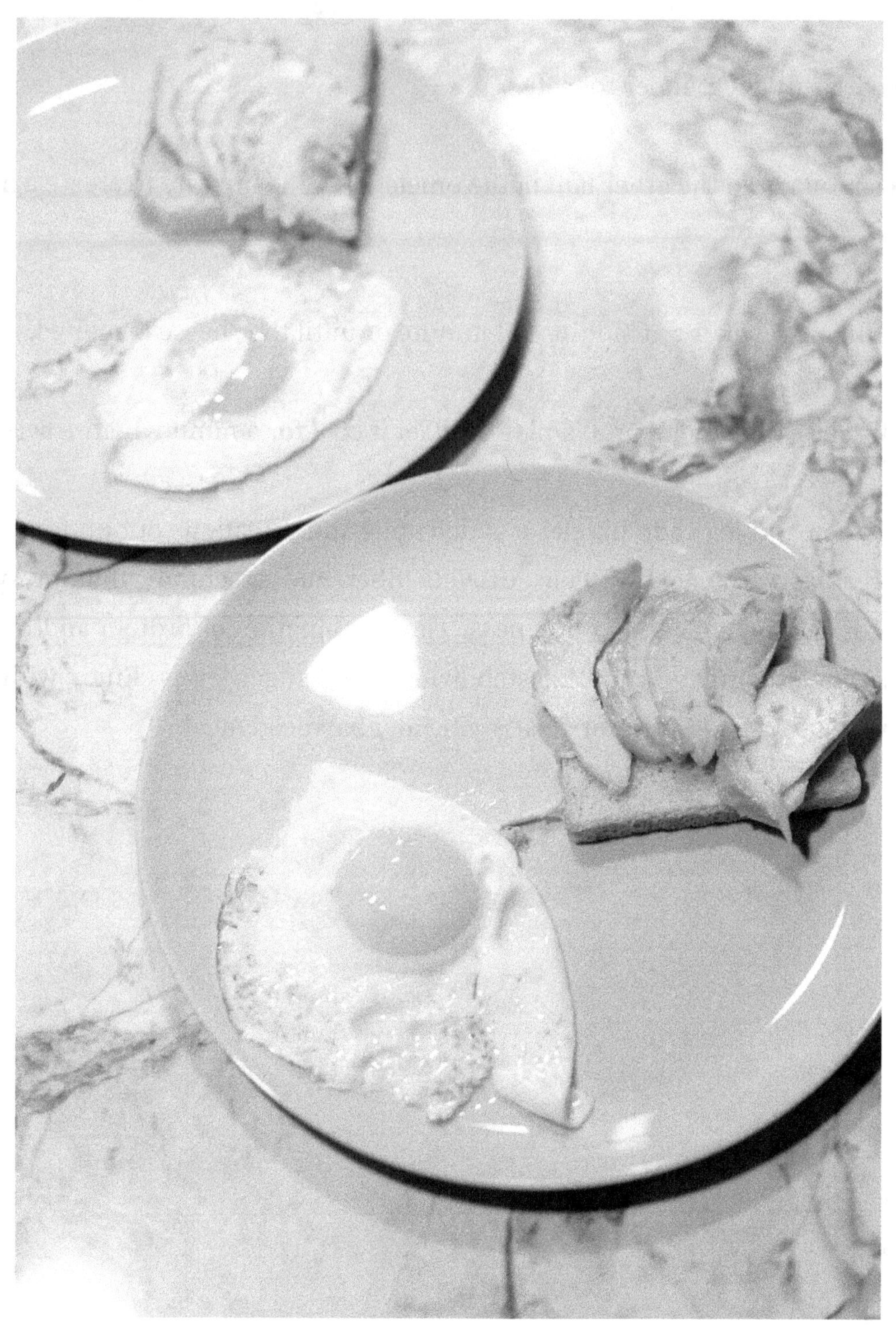

Zucchini and Feta Cheese Frittata

Ingredients:

- 2 medium-sized zucchinis, thinly sliced

- 6 eggs

- 1/4 cup crumbled feta cheese

- 1/4 cup low-fat milk

- 1 tablespoon olive oil

- 1 teaspoon dried oregano

- Salt and pepper to taste

Instructions:

1. Preheat your oven to 375°F (190°C).

2. In a large non-stick oven-safe skillet, heat the olive oil over medium heat.

3. Add the zucchini slices and sauté for 2-3 minutes, until slightly softened.

4. In a separate bowl, beat the eggs with the milk, dried oregano, and a pinch of salt and pepper.

5. Pour the egg mixture into the skillet with the zucchini and give it a quick stir to evenly distribute the zucchini.

6. Let the mixture cook for 3-4 minutes, until the edges are set but the center is still slightly runny.

7. Sprinkle the crumbled feta cheese on top of the frittata.

8. Transfer the skillet to the oven and bake for 12-15 minutes, until the frittata is set and the top is slightly golden.

9. Remove from the oven and let it cool for 2-3 minutes before serving.

10. Use a spatula to slide the frittata onto a cutting board.

11. Cut into 4 pieces and serve warm.

Tips:

- You can add other low-carb vegetables such as bell peppers or spinach to the frittata for added flavor and nutrients.
- Serve with a side salad or whole wheat toast for a complete meal.
- Leftovers can be stored in the refrigerator for up to 3 days and reheated in the microwave or on the stovetop.

Related Book Type 1 Diabetes Cookbook For Kids, Teens, Women, Men And Adults **By Caroline Johnson**

Whole Wheat Banana Pancakes

Ingredients:

- 1 large ripe banana
- 1 cup whole wheat flour
- 1 teaspoon baking powder
- 1/4 teaspoon salt
- 1/4 teaspoon ground cinnamon
- 1/2 cup unsweetened almond milk
- 1 egg
- 1 tablespoon honey
- 1 tablespoon coconut oil
- Optional toppings: sugar-free syrup, fresh berries

Instructions:

1. In a mixing bowl, mash the ripe banana until smooth.
2. Add in the whole wheat flour, baking powder, salt, and ground cinnamon. Mix well.
3. In a separate bowl, whisk together the almond milk, egg, honey, and coconut oil.
4. Pour the wet mixture into the dry mixture and stir until well combined.
5. Let the batter rest for 5 minutes.
6. Heat a non-stick pan or griddle over medium heat.
7. Using a measuring cup or ladle, pour 1/4 cup of batter onto the pan for each pancake.
8. Cook for about 2-3 minutes on each side, flipping when bubbles start to form.
9. Once cooked, remove from the pan and set aside on a plate. Repeat until all the batter is used up.
10. Serve the pancakes warm with your preferred toppings, such as sugar-free syrup and fresh berries.

Tips:

- To add more flavor, you can also add 1/4 teaspoon of vanilla extract to the batter.
- If the batter is too thick, you can add a little bit of extra almond milk to thin it out.

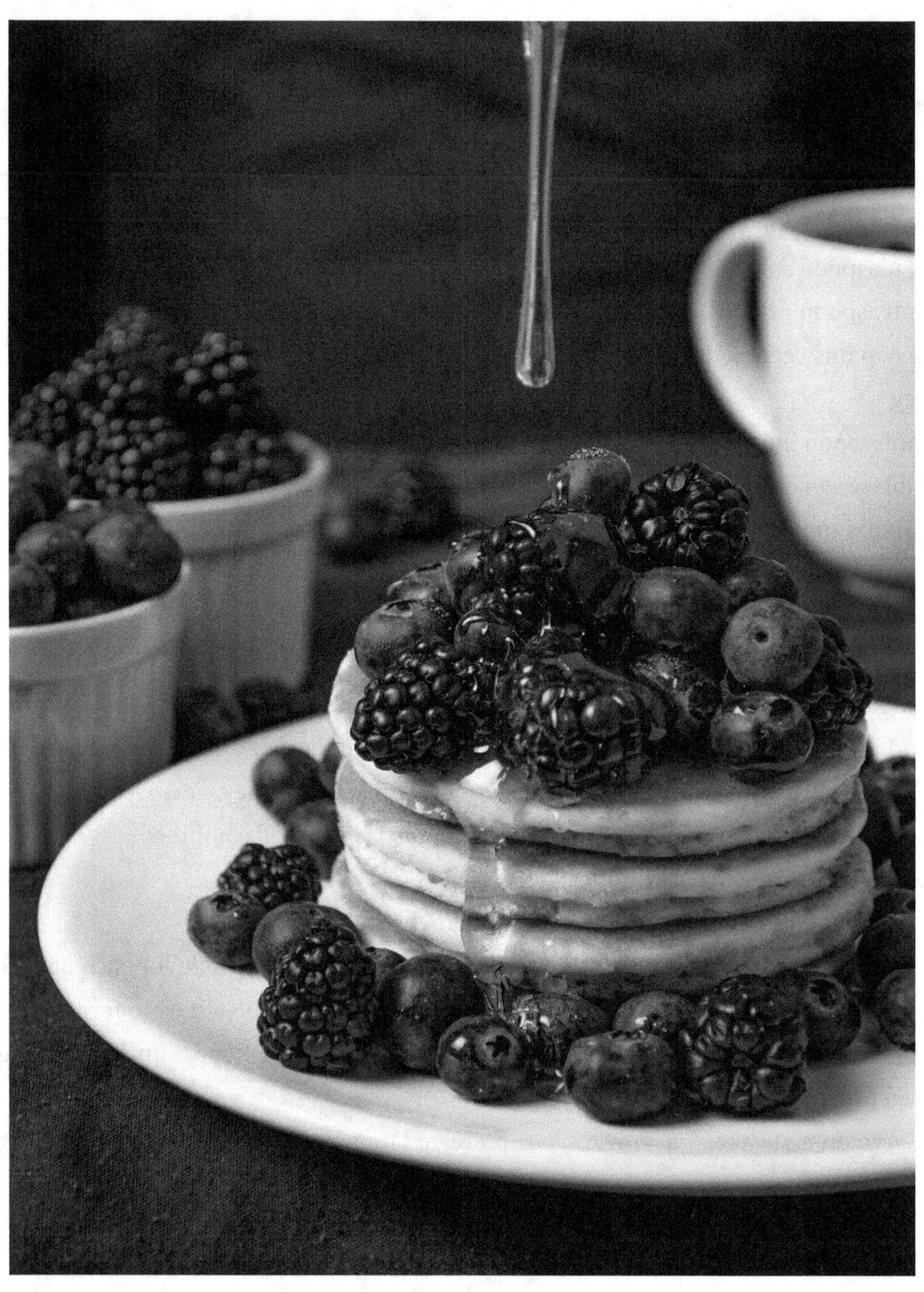

- Make sure to use a non-stick pan or cooking spray to prevent the pancakes from sticking.

- These pancakes are best consumed immediately, but can also be stored in an airtight container in the fridge for up to 3 days.

- You can also double or triple the recipe and freeze the remaining pancakes for future breakfasts.

Nutritional Information:

Serving size: 1 pancake (without toppings)

Calories: 110

Carbohydrates: 18g

Protein: 3g

Fat: 3g

Sodium: 167mg

Fiber: 2g

Sugar: 4g

Low Carb Breakfast Bowl

The low carb diet has been gaining popularity for its ability to help with weight loss and improve overall health. As a type 2 diabetes patient, breakfast can be a struggle as traditional breakfast options like toast, cereal, and pancakes are off the table. However, with a little creativity and some delicious ingredients, a low carb breakfast bowl can make for a satisfying and nutritious morning meal.

Ingredients:

- 2 eggs
- 1/2 avocado, sliced
- 1 small tomato, diced
- 1 cup spinach, chopped
- 1/4 cup shredded cheddar cheese
- 2 strips of bacon, cooked and crumbled
- Salt and pepper to taste

Instructions:

1. Start by cooking the eggs to your preference. You can either scramble them in a pan or cook them sunny side up. Set aside once cooked.

2. In a mixing bowl, combine the avocado, tomato, spinach, and cheddar cheese. Toss together to make a flavorful and colorful salad.

3. Place the salad mixture at the bottom of a bowl to create a base for your breakfast bowl.

4. Top the salad with the cooked eggs and sprinkle with salt and pepper to taste.

5. Finally, add the crumbled bacon on top for a crispy and savory addition to your low carb breakfast bowl.

This breakfast bowl is not only low in carbs, but it is also packed with protein, healthy fats, and essential vitamins and minerals. The eggs provide a hearty source of protein to keep you feeling full and satisfied until your next meal. Avocado is a great source of healthy fats, which are essential for brain function and can also help to keep you feeling full. The tomatoes and spinach add a powerful dose of vitamins and antioxidants to your breakfast bowl.

For those following a low carb diet, this breakfast bowl is a perfect way to start your day. It is easy to prepare and is customizable based on your personal preferences and dietary restrictions. For those who do not eat bacon, it can easily be replaced with turkey bacon or omitted altogether. You can also add in other vegetables like bell peppers, onions, or mushrooms to add even more flavor and nutrients.

In addition to being a great breakfast option, this low carb breakfast bowl can also be enjoyed as a light and healthy lunch or dinner. It is a versatile and delicious meal that will leave you feeling energized and satisfied without the carb overload. Give it a try and see for yourself how delicious and nutritious a low carb breakfast bowl can be!

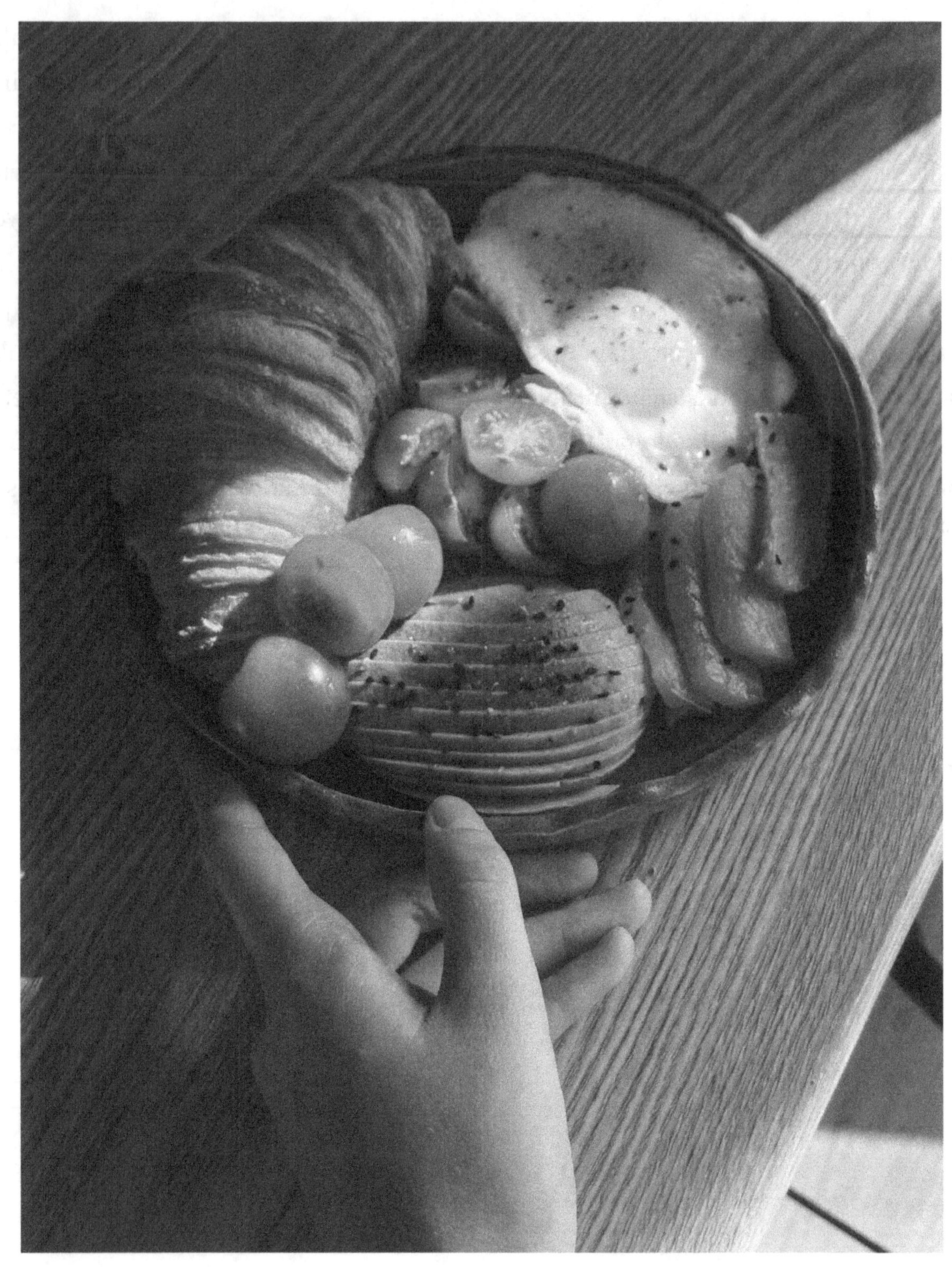

Overnight Oats with Berries

Ingredients:

- 1/2 cup rolled oats

- 1/2 cup unsweetened almond milk

- 1/4 cup plain Greek yogurt

- 1/4 cup fresh berries (raspberries, blueberries, or strawberries)

- 1 tbsp chia seeds

- 1 tsp honey (optional)

- 1 tsp cinnamon (optional)

Instructions:

1. In a mason jar or bowl, mix the rolled oats, almond milk, Greek yogurt, and chia seeds. If you would like your oats to be sweeter, you can add 1 tsp of honey at this point.

2. Cover the jar/bowl and place it in the refrigerator overnight. This allows the oats to soften and the flavors to develop.

3. In the morning, take the jar/bowl out of the refrigerator and stir the oats mixture.

4. Add in the fresh berries of your choice and gently mix them in.

5. If desired, sprinkle a tsp of cinnamon on top for added flavor and health benefits.

6. Enjoy your delicious and healthy overnight oat and berries for breakfast!

Nutritional information:
Serving size: 1 jar/bowl
Calories: 300
Carbohydrates: 40g
Protein: 11g
Fat: 10g

Fiber: 8g

Oats are a great source of fiber and help regulate blood sugar levels. The chia seeds are also high in fiber and contain healthy fats that are beneficial for type 2 diabetes patients. The Greek yogurt adds protein and the berries provide natural sweetness and antioxidants. The addition of cinnamon can help improve insulin sensitivity and regulate blood sugar levels. This recipe is a filling and nutritious breakfast option for type 2 diabetes patients.

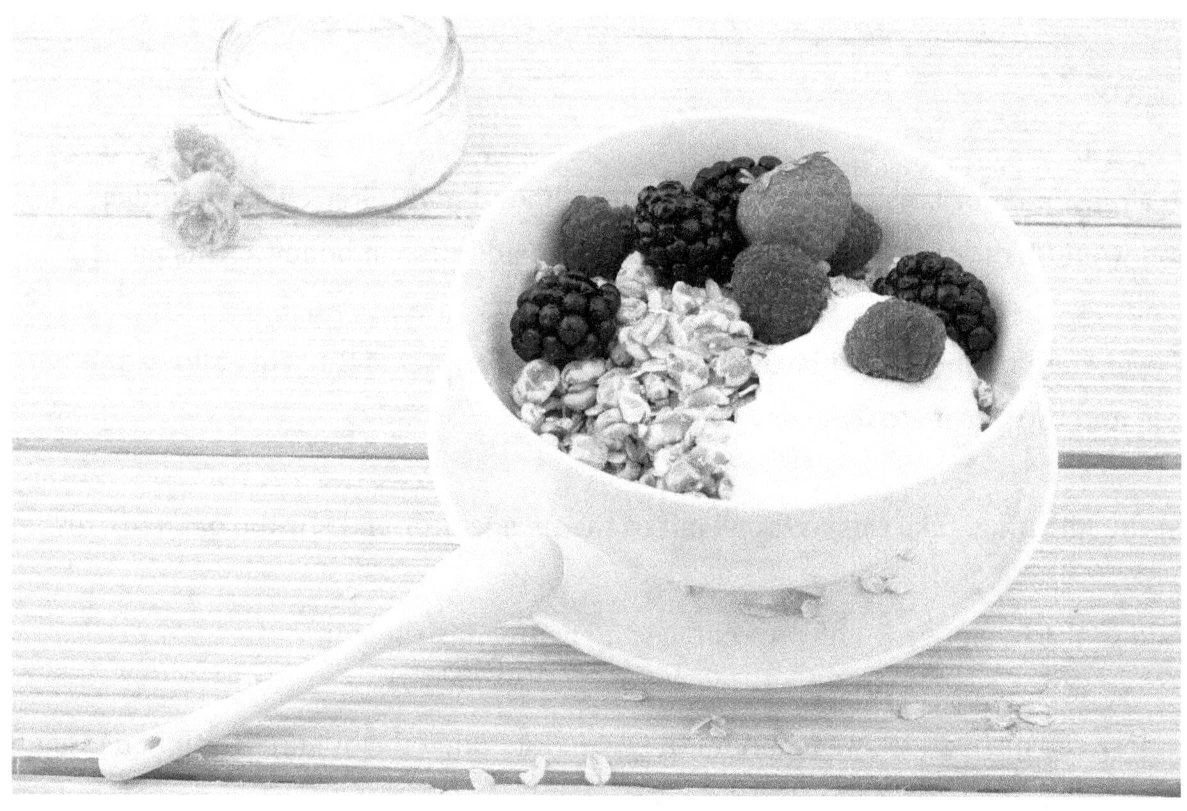

Quinoa and Black Bean Salad

Ingredients:

- 1 cup uncooked quinoa
- 1 can black beans, rinsed and drained
- 1 red bell pepper, diced
- 1 small red onion, finely diced
- 1/4 cup fresh cilantro, chopped
- 1 avocado, diced
- 1/4 cup extra virgin olive oil
- Juice of 1 lime
- 1 garlic clove, minced
- Salt and black pepper to taste

Instructions:

1. Rinse the quinoa and drain it well. In a small saucepan, bring 2 cups of water to a boil. Add the quinoa, reduce the heat to low, and cover. Let the quinoa simmer for about 15 minutes, or until all the water is absorbed and the quinoa is tender. Fluff with a fork and let it cool down.

2. In a small bowl, mix together the extra virgin olive oil, lime juice, minced garlic, and a pinch of salt and black pepper to make the dressing.

3. In a large mixing bowl, add the cooked quinoa, black beans, diced red pepper, red onion, and chopped cilantro. Toss everything together.

4. Pour the dressing over the quinoa and bean mixture and stir it well.

5. Gently fold in the diced avocado.

6. Taste the salad and adjust the seasoning if needed.

7. Refrigerate the salad for at least 30 minutes before serving to allow the flavors to fully infuse together.

8. Garnish with some extra cilantro before serving if desired.

Quinoa and Black Bean Salad is a healthy and tasty option for type 2 diabetes patients, as it is packed with fiber, protein, and healthy fats. It can be enjoyed as a light lunch or served as a side dish with your favorite protein. Make sure to stick to portion control and pair it with a balanced meal to manage your blood sugar levels. Enjoy!

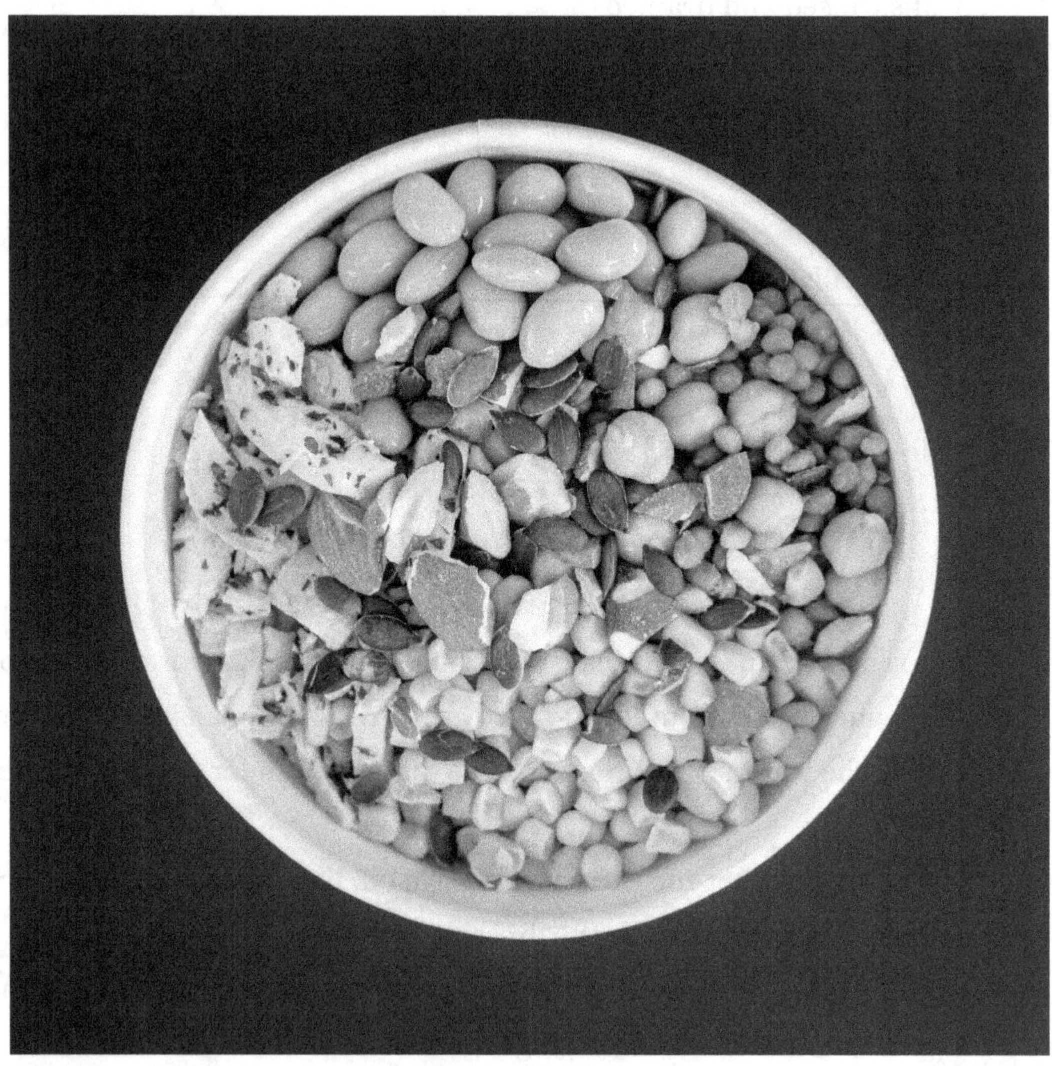

Grilled Chicken and Vegetable Wrap

Ingredients:

- 4 whole wheat tortillas
- 1 lb boneless, skinless chicken breast
- 1 small onion, sliced
- 1 red bell pepper, sliced
- 1 green bell pepper, sliced
- 1 zucchini, sliced
- 1 yellow squash, sliced
- 2 cloves garlic, minced
- 1 tsp olive oil
- 1 tsp dried oregano
- 1 tsp dried basil
- Salt and pepper, to taste
- 1 tbsp balsamic vinegar
- 4 tbsp reduced-fat cream cheese
- 2 cups spinach

Instructions:

1. Begin by marinating the chicken breast with the minced garlic, dried oregano, dried basil, salt, pepper, and balsamic vinegar. Let it sit for 15 minutes.

2. Meanwhile, preheat a grill or a grill pan to medium-high heat.

3. Grill the marinated chicken breast for about 6-7 minutes on each side, or until it's fully cooked.

4. In a separate pan, heat the olive oil over medium-high heat. Add the sliced onions, bell peppers, zucchini, and squash. Saute for about 5 minutes, or until the vegetables are tender.

5. Warm the tortillas on the grill for about 30 seconds on each side.

6. Spread 1 tablespoon of reduced-fat cream cheese on each tortilla.

7. Place a handful of spinach on top of the cream cheese.

8. Slice the grilled chicken breast into thin strips and place on top of the spinach.

9. Add the sautéed vegetables on top of the chicken.

10. Roll up the tortilla tightly, tucking in the ends to prevent the filling from falling out.

11. Place the wrapped tortillas on the grill for an additional 1-2 minutes on each side to heat through.

12. Serve hot and enjoy your delicious and healthy Grilled Chicken and Vegetable Wraps.

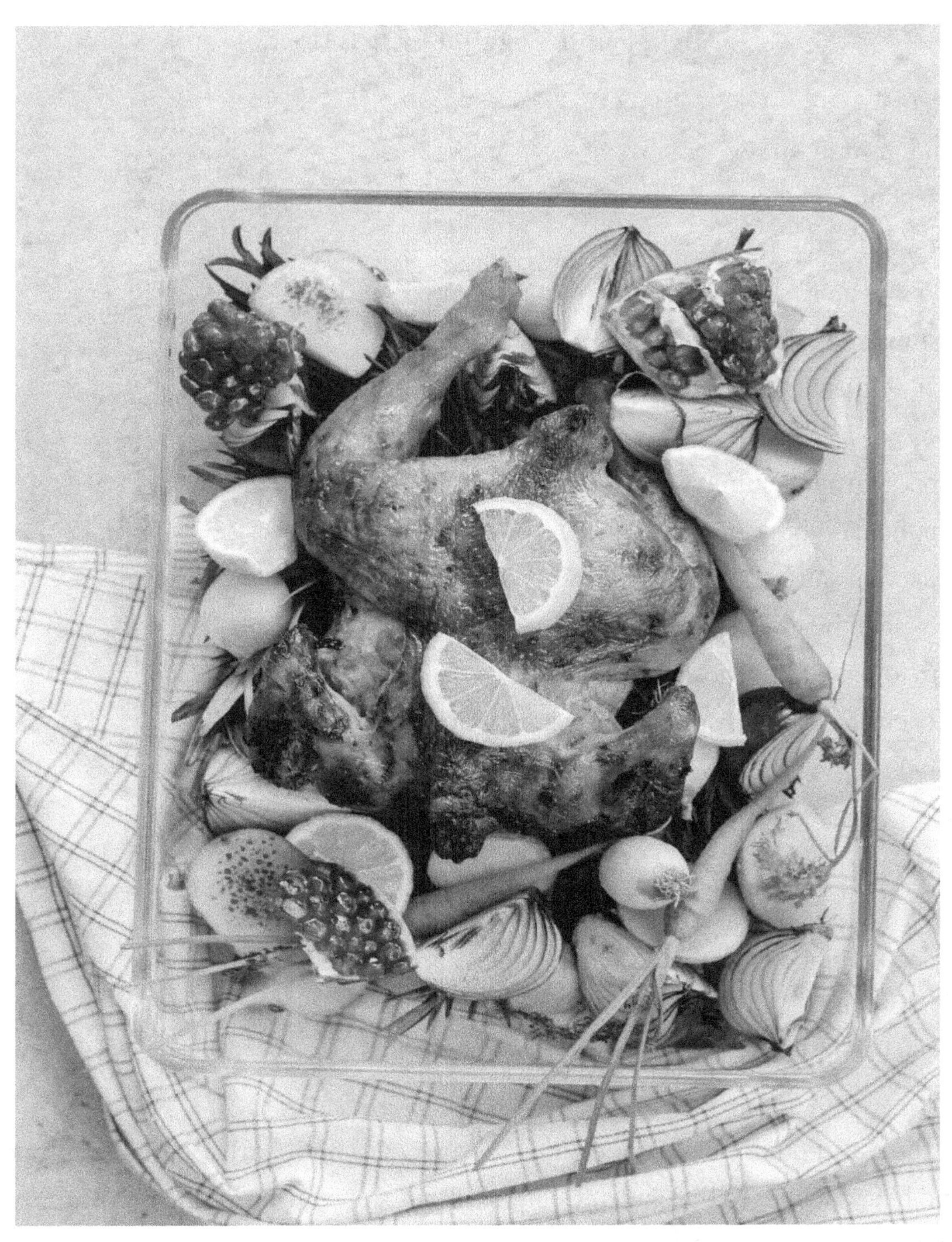

Turkey and Veggie Lettuce Wraps

Ingredients:
- 1 pound ground turkey
- 1 tablespoon olive oil
- 1/2 onion, diced
- 1 red bell pepper, diced
- 1 cup mushrooms, sliced
- 1 zucchini, diced
- 2 cloves garlic, minced
- 1 teaspoon ground cumin
- 1 teaspoon chili powder
- 1/2 teaspoon salt
- 1/2 teaspoon black pepper
- 1/4 cup low-sodium chicken broth
- 8 large lettuce leaves (romaine or iceberg work best)
- Optional toppings: shredded cheese, avocado, salsa, diced tomatoes

Instructions:

1. In a large skillet, heat 1 tablespoon of olive oil over medium heat.

2. Add the ground turkey, breaking it up with a wooden spoon, and cook until browned.

3. Add the diced onion, bell pepper, mushrooms, zucchini, garlic, cumin, chili powder, salt, and black pepper to the skillet. Cook for about 5 minutes, stirring occasionally, until the vegetables are softened.

4. Pour in the chicken broth and continue to cook for another 5 minutes.

5. While the turkey and veggies are cooking, wash and dry the lettuce leaves.

6. Once the turkey is fully cooked and the vegetables are tender, turn off the heat and let the mixture cool for a few minutes.

7. Assemble the lettuce wraps by placing a few spoonfuls of the turkey and veggie mixture onto a lettuce leaf and rolling it up like a taco.

8. Serve the wraps with optional toppings such as shredded cheese, avocado, salsa, or diced tomatoes.

9. Enjoy your healthy and delicious Turkey and Veggie Lettuce Wraps! Store any leftovers in the refrigerator for up to 3 days.

Tips:
- For a vegetarian option, substitute the ground turkey with tofu or add extra vegetables such as diced carrots or corn.
- To lower the sodium content, use low-sodium chicken broth and omit the salt.
- You can also add a bit of heat to the wraps by adding a dash of hot sauce or red pepper flakes.
- These lettuce wraps are packed with fiber and protein, making them a great option for a balanced and nutritious meal for type 2 diabetes patients. Enjoy!

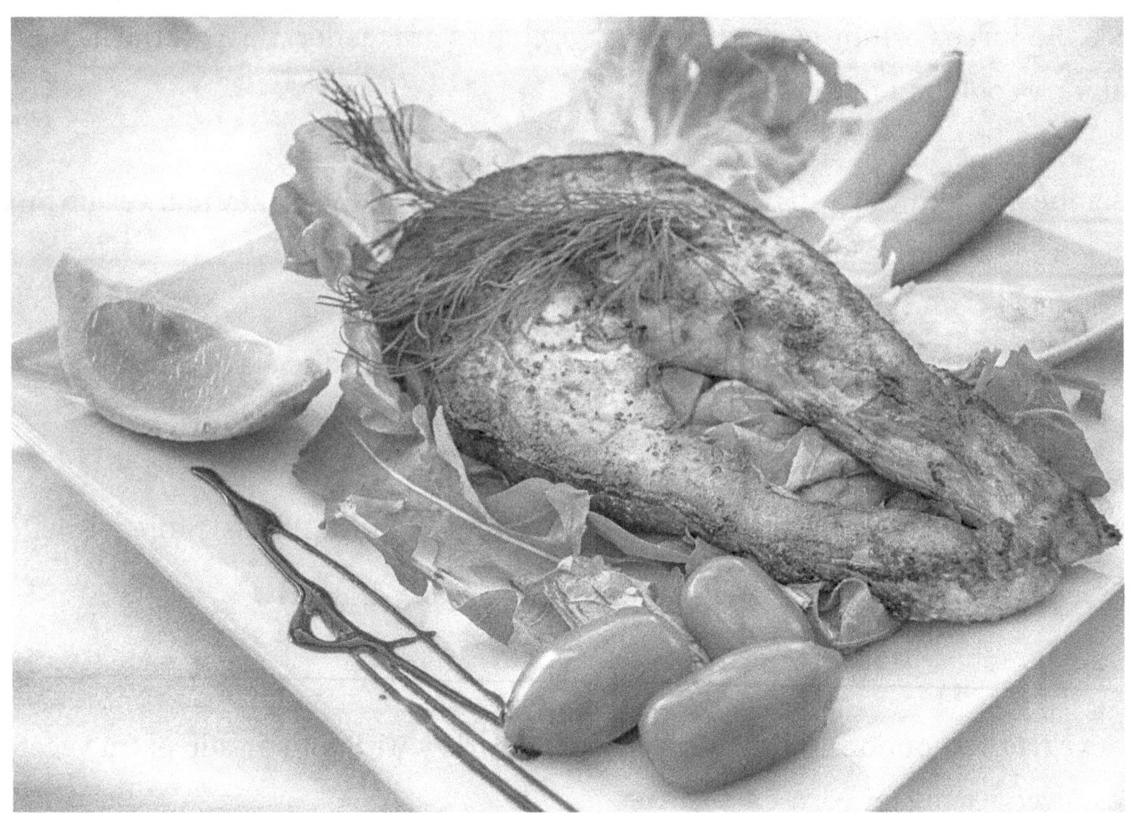

Visit Caroline Johnson Author Central page for more health books

Roasted Vegetable and Hummus Sandwich

Ingredients:
- 1 medium zucchini
- 1 medium eggplant
- 1 small red bell pepper
- 1 small yellow bell pepper
- 1 small red onion
- 2 tablespoons olive oil
- Salt and pepper to taste
- 4 slices of whole grain bread
- 1/2 cup hummus
- 1/4 cup crumbled feta cheese
- Fresh basil leaves (optional)

Instructions:

1. Preheat your oven to 400°F (200°C).

2. Wash and dry the zucchini, eggplant, bell peppers, and onion. Cut the zucchini and eggplant into thin round slices, and the bell peppers and onion into thin strips.

3. Place the vegetables on a baking sheet and drizzle with olive oil. Toss to coat evenly. Season with salt and pepper to taste.

4. Roast the vegetables for 20-25 minutes, or until they are tender and slightly golden.

5. While the vegetables are roasting, toast the bread slices in a toaster or on a skillet until lightly browned.

6. Once the vegetables are done, take them out of the oven and let them cool for a few minutes.

7. Spread a generous amount of hummus on each slice of toasted bread.

8. Layer the roasted vegetables evenly on top of the hummus. You can also add some crumbled feta cheese and fresh basil leaves for extra flavor and texture.

9. Place the other slice of bread on top to make a sandwich.

10. Cut the sandwich in half and enjoy!

This roasted vegetable and hummus sandwich is high in fiber and protein, making it a great option for type 2 diabetes patients. It is also packed with nutrients from the roasted vegetables and is a delicious and filling meal. Serve with a side of fresh fruit for a complete and balanced meal. Enjoy!

Greek Yogurt Chicken Salad

Ingredients:
- 1 cup cooked and shredded chicken breast
- 1/2 cup plain Greek yogurt
- 1/4 cup diced celery
- 1/4 cup diced red onion
- 1/4 cup diced cucumber
- 1/4 cup halved cherry tomatoes
- 1 tablespoon chopped fresh dill
- Juice of 1/2 lemon
- Salt and pepper to taste

Instructions:

1. In a medium sized bowl, mix together the cooked and shredded chicken breast, Greek yogurt, celery, red onion, cucumber, cherry tomatoes, dill, lemon juice, and salt and pepper.

2. Taste and adjust seasoning as desired. If you prefer a creamier texture, you can add more Greek yogurt.

3. Cover the bowl and place in the refrigerator for at least 30 minutes to allow the flavors to meld together.

4. Serve the Greek Yogurt Chicken Salad on top of a bed of lettuce or in a whole wheat pita for a delicious and healthy meal.

Baked Salmon with Lemon and Herbs

Ingredients:

- 4 salmon fillets

- 1 lemon

- 2 tablespoons of olive oil

- Salt and pepper

- 1 teaspoon of dried parsley

- 1 teaspoon of dried dill

- 1 teaspoon of dried thyme

- 1 teaspoon of garlic powder

- 1 teaspoon of onion powder

Instructions:

1. Preheat your oven to 375°F (190°C).

2. Rinse the salmon fillets and pat them dry with paper towels. Place them in a baking dish coated with cooking spray.

3. In a small bowl, mix together the olive oil, dried parsley, dill, thyme, garlic powder, onion powder, and a pinch of salt and pepper.

4. Brush the herbed oil mixture onto the salmon fillets, making sure to cover them evenly.

5. Slice the lemon into thin, round pieces and place them on top of the salmon fillets.

6. Cover the dish with foil and bake for 15-20 minutes, or until the salmon is opaque and flakes easily with a fork.

7. Remove the foil for the last 5 minutes of cooking to allow the top of the salmon to brown slightly.

8. Take the salmon out of the oven and let it rest for a few minutes before serving.

9. Serve the baked salmon with lemon and herbs with your choice of sides, such as steamed vegetables or a small side salad.

This dish is both delicious and suitable for type 2 diabetes patients as it avoids high-sugar or high-carbohydrate ingredients and includes healthy herbs and oils. The fiber and essential fatty acids found in the salmon are beneficial for managing blood sugar levels. Enjoy this easy, flavorful and diabetes-friendly meal!

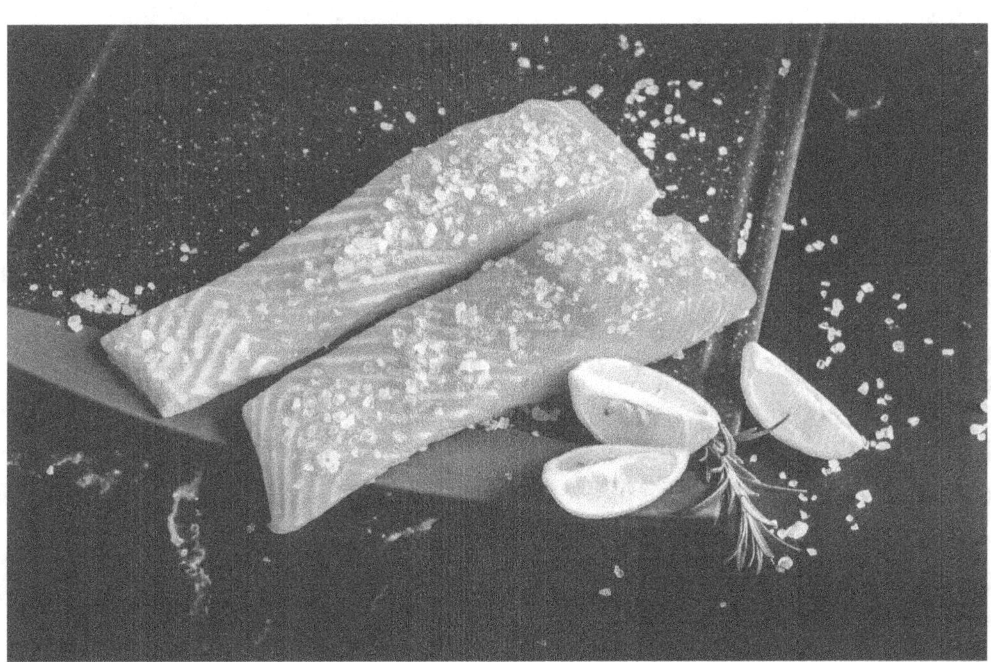

Cauliflower Fried Rice

Ingredients:

- 1 head of cauliflower

- 1 tablespoon olive oil

- 1 small onion, diced

- 2 cloves of garlic, minced

- 1 cup of mixed vegetables (carrots, peas, corn)

- 2 eggs

- 2 tablespoons low-sodium soy sauce

- 1 teaspoon ginger, minced

- Salt and pepper to taste

Instructions:

1. Begin by washing and drying the head of cauliflower. Cut it into small florets and discard the stems. Place the florets in a food processor and pulse until it resembles rice-like grains.

2. Heat a large skillet or wok over medium heat and add the olive oil. Once hot, add the diced onion and minced garlic. Stir and cook for 2-3 minutes until the onions become translucent.

3. Add the mixed vegetables to the skillet and cook for an additional 2-3 minutes.

4. Move the vegetables to one side of the skillet and crack the two eggs on the other side. Let them cook for a minute or two and then scramble them with a spatula, combining them with the vegetables.

5. Add the riced cauliflower, low-sodium soy sauce, and minced ginger to the skillet. Season with salt and pepper to taste. Stir well to combine all the ingredients.

6. Cook for 5-7 minutes, stirring occasionally, until the cauliflower rice is tender.

7. Serve hot and enjoy your delicious and healthy Cauliflower Fried Rice! You can top it with some chopped scallions or a sprinkle of sesame seeds if desired.

This recipe includes low-carb, low-glycemic index ingredients that are suitable for a type 2 diabetes diet. It is a great alternative to traditional fried rice and provides a good source of fiber and nutrients. Enjoy as a main dish or as a side with lean protein such as grilled chicken or fish.

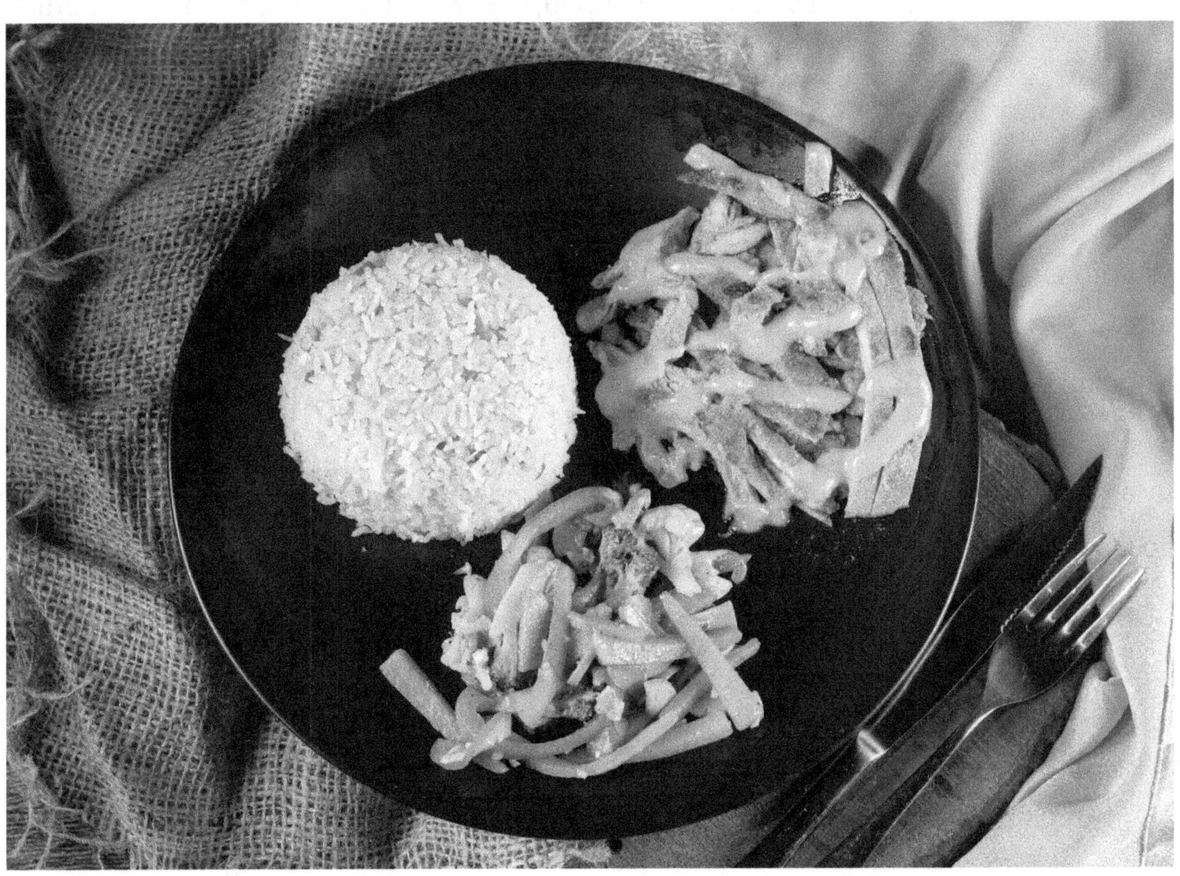

Balsamic Glazed Chicken with Roasted Vegetables

Ingredients:
- 4 boneless, skinless chicken breasts
- 1/4 cup balsamic vinegar
- 1/4 cup olive oil
- 1 tbsp honey
- 1 tsp Dijon mustard
- 1 tsp minced garlic
- Salt and pepper, to taste
- 4 cups of assorted vegetables (such as bell peppers, zucchini, mushrooms, and onions), chopped
- Cooking spray
- Fresh parsley for garnish (optional)

Instructions:

1. Preheat your oven to 400°F (200°C).

2. In a small bowl, mix together the balsamic vinegar, olive oil, honey, Dijon mustard, minced garlic, and a sprinkle of salt and pepper. This will be the marinade for your chicken.

3. Place the chicken breasts in a large zip-top bag and pour the marinade over them. Squeeze out any excess air from the bag and seal. Massage the marinade onto the chicken to evenly coat them. Let it marinate in the fridge for at least 30 minutes, or up to 2 hours.

4. After marinating, take the chicken out of the fridge and let it sit at room temperature for 10-15 minutes.

5. Meanwhile, prepare your vegetables. Chop them into bite-sized pieces and place them in a single layer on a baking sheet lined with parchment paper.

6. Spray the vegetables with cooking spray and sprinkle with salt and pepper.

7. Remove the chicken from the marinade and place them on the baking sheet with the vegetables.

8. Bake in the oven for 25-30 minutes, or until the chicken is cooked through and the veggies are tender. The chicken should have an internal temperature of 165°F (74°C) when done.

9. While the chicken and vegetables are cooking, pour the remaining marinade into a small saucepan and bring it to a boil. Let it simmer for a few minutes until it thickens into a glaze.

10. Once the chicken and vegetables are done, brush the glaze over the chicken.

11. Serve the Balsamic Glazed Chicken with Roasted Vegetables hot, garnished with fresh parsley if desired.

Enjoy your delicious and diabetes-friendly meal! For best results, pair it with a side of brown rice or quinoa for a balanced and filling meal.

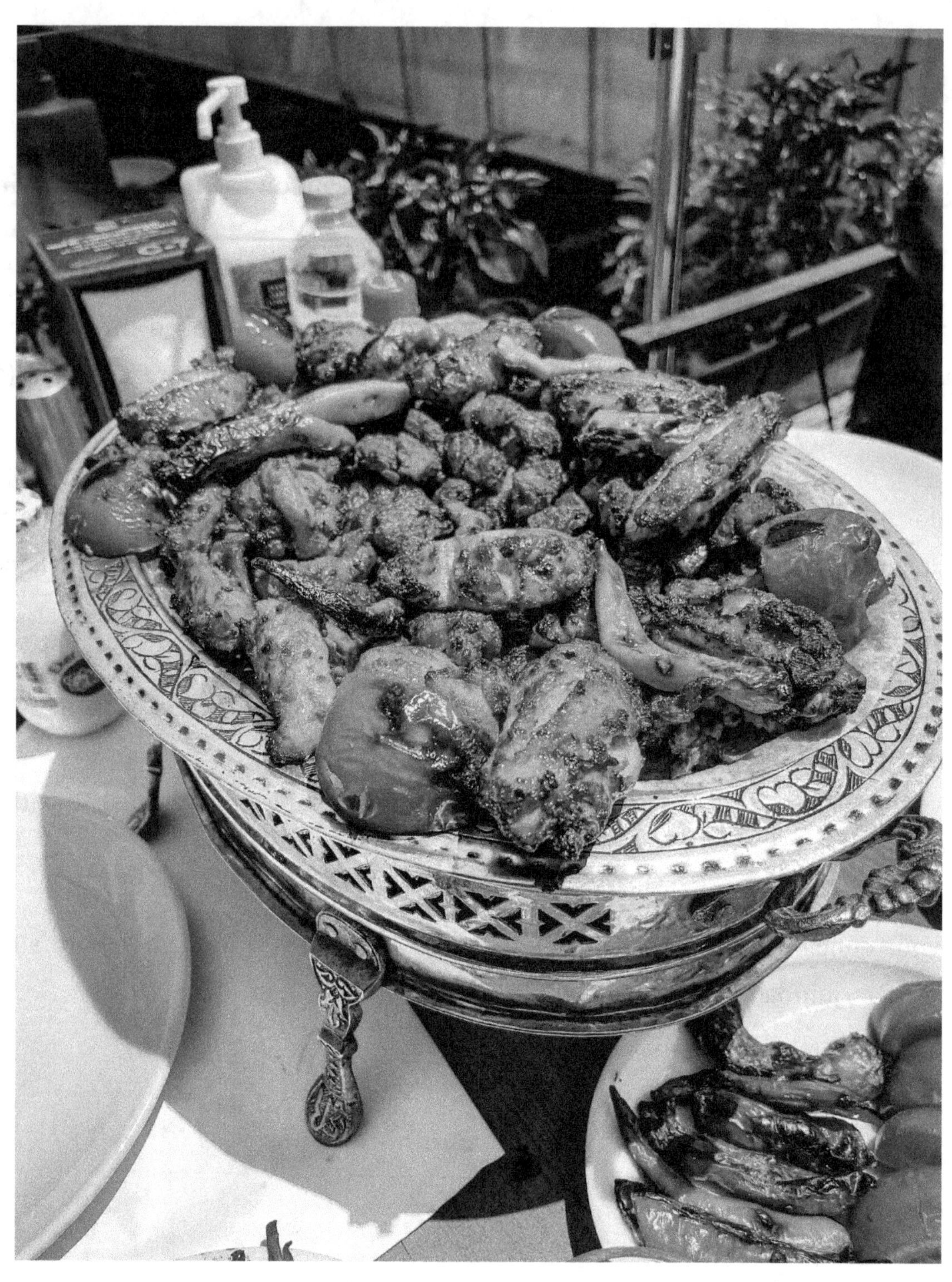

Turkey and Vegetable Stir-Fry

Ingredients:

- 1 pound turkey breast, cut into thin strips
- 2 tablespoons olive oil
- 1 onion, sliced
- 2 cloves of garlic, minced
- 1 cup broccoli florets
- 1 red bell pepper, sliced
- 1 cup sugar snap peas
- 1 cup mushrooms, sliced
- 2 cups spinach
- 2 tablespoons low-sodium soy sauce
- 1 tablespoon honey
- 1 teaspoon ginger, minced
- 1 teaspoon red pepper flakes (optional)
- Salt and pepper to taste
- Brown rice, cooked (optional)

Instructions:

1. In a large skillet or wok, heat 1 tablespoon of olive oil over medium-high heat. Add the turkey strips and cook until they are no longer pink, about 5-6 minutes. Remove the turkey from the skillet and set aside.

2. In the same skillet, add the remaining tablespoon of olive oil. Add the onion and garlic, and sauté for 2-3 minutes until they become fragrant.

3. Add the broccoli florets, red bell pepper, sugar snap peas, and mushrooms to the skillet. Stir-fry for 4-5 minutes until the vegetables become tender but still retain their crunch.

4. Add the spinach to the skillet and cook until it wilts, about 2-3 minutes.

5. In a small bowl, mix together the low-sodium soy sauce, honey, ginger, red pepper flakes (if using), and a pinch of salt and pepper.

6. Pour the sauce over the vegetables in the skillet and stir to coat evenly.

7. Add the cooked turkey back to the skillet and stir to combine with the vegetables and sauce. Cook for an additional 2-3 minutes until everything is heated through.

8. Serve the stir-fry with brown rice, if desired. Enjoy your healthy and delicious Turkey and Vegetable Stir-Fry!

Visit Caroline Johnson Author Central page for more health books

Stuffed Bell Peppers

Ingredients:

-4 large bell peppers

-1 tablespoon of olive oil

-1 small onion, chopped

-1 clove of garlic, minced

-1 pound of lean ground turkey or chicken

-1 cup of cooked brown rice

-1/2 cup of low-fat shredded cheese

-1 teaspoon of dried oregano

-1 teaspoon of dried basil

-1/2 teaspoon of salt

-1/4 teaspoon of black pepper

-1 can (14.5 ounces) of low-sodium diced tomatoes

-1/4 cup of low-sodium chicken broth

Instructions:

1. Preheat your oven to 375°F (190°C).

2. Cut off the tops of the bell peppers and remove the seeds and membranes. Rinse them thoroughly and set them aside.

3. In a large skillet, heat the olive oil over medium heat. Add the chopped onions and minced garlic. Cook for 2-3 minutes, stirring occasionally, until they become translucent.

4. Add the ground turkey or chicken to the skillet and cook until it is no longer pink, around 5-7 minutes.

5. Stir in the cooked brown rice, dried oregano, dried basil, salt, and black pepper. Cook for an additional 2-3 minutes.

6. Add the diced tomatoes and chicken broth to the skillet and let it simmer for 5 minutes, until the liquid has reduced.

7. Stuff the mixture into the hollowed-out bell peppers and place them in a baking dish.

8. Bake the stuffed bell peppers for 30-35 minutes, until the peppers are tender.

9. Sprinkle the shredded cheese on top of the peppers and bake for an additional 5 minutes until the cheese is melted.

10. Remove from the oven and let it cool for a few minutes before serving. Enjoy your delicious and healthy Stuffed Bell Peppers!

Tips:

- You can use any color of bell peppers for this recipe, but red or yellow peppers tend to be sweeter and have more nutrients.

- If you prefer a vegetarian option, you can substitute the ground turkey or chicken with tofu or quinoa.

- To save time, you can use pre-cooked brown rice instead of cooking it from scratch.

- This recipe can be made ahead of time and stored in the fridge for up to 2 days. Just reheat in the oven or microwave before serving.

Roasted Chickpeas

Ingredients:

- 1 can of chickpeas, drained and rinsed

- 1 tablespoon of olive oil

- 1 teaspoon of garlic powder

- 1 teaspoon of paprika

- 1/2 teaspoon of cumin

- 1/4 teaspoon of salt

- 1/4 teaspoon of black pepper

Instructions:

1. Preheat your oven to 400 degrees Fahrenheit (200 degrees Celsius).

2. In a mixing bowl, combine the drained and rinsed chickpeas with olive oil, garlic powder, paprika, cumin, salt, and black pepper. Mix well until the chickpeas are evenly coated.

3. Spread the chickpeas in a single layer on a baking sheet lined with parchment paper.

4. Place the baking sheet in the preheated oven and bake for 20-25 minutes, stirring the chickpeas halfway through the cooking time. This will ensure that they are evenly roasted.

5. After 20-25 minutes, remove the baking sheet from the oven and let the chickpeas cool down for a few minutes.

6. Serve the roasted chickpeas as a healthy and delicious snack for your type 2 diabetes diet. You can also add them to salads or use them as a topping for soups and stews.

Tip: You can experiment with different spices and herbs to flavor your roasted chickpeas, such as chili powder, curry powder, or Italian seasoning. Just be mindful of the sodium content in pre-made spice blends and adjust the amount of salt accordingly. Enjoy!

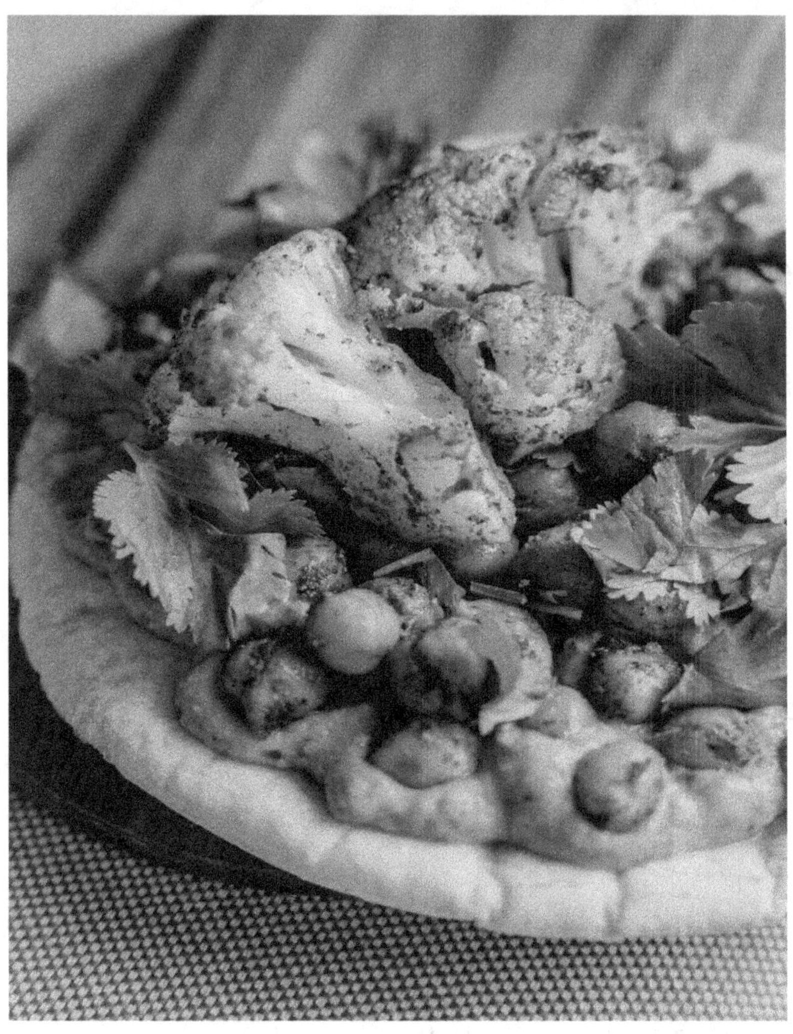

Spiced Nuts

Ingredients:

- 2 cups mixed unsalted nuts (almonds, walnuts, cashews, etc.)
- 1 tablespoon olive oil
- 1 tablespoon honey
- 1 teaspoon ground cinnamon
- 1/4 teaspoon ground ginger
- 1/4 teaspoon ground nutmeg
- 1/4 teaspoon ground cloves
- 1/4 teaspoon salt
- Non-stick cooking spray

Instructions:

1. Preheat your oven to 350 degrees Fahrenheit.

2. In a small bowl, mix together the olive oil, honey, ground cinnamon, ground ginger, ground nutmeg, ground cloves, and salt. Set aside.

3. Place the mixed nuts in a mixing bowl. Pour the spice mixture over the nuts and toss well until all the nuts are evenly coated.

4. Spray a baking sheet with non-stick cooking spray. Spread the spiced nuts in a single layer on the baking sheet.

5. Bake in the preheated oven for 10-12 minutes, stirring occasionally, until the nuts are lightly toasted.

6. Remove the baking sheet from the oven and let the spiced nuts cool for a few minutes.

7. Once cooled, transfer the spiced nuts to an airtight container and store in a cool, dry place. They can be stored for up to two weeks.

8. Serve the spiced nuts as a snack on their own or add them to salads or yogurt for some extra crunch and flavor.

Notes:
- This recipe makes approximately 2 cups of spiced nuts.
- You can adjust the amount of spices and honey according to your taste preference, but keep in mind that excessive amounts of sugar may not be suitable for a type 2 diabetes patient.
- Avoid using pre-packaged mixed nuts that may contain added salt, sugar or unhealthy oils.
- These spiced nuts are high in healthy fats, protein, and fiber, making them a great snack option for type 2 diabetes patients. However, it is important to monitor portion sizes to avoid overeating.
- Store leftover spiced nuts in an airtight container in the fridge for longer storage. They can be reheated in the oven for a few minutes before serving for a fresh, warm snack.

Veggie and Hummus Platter

Ingredients:
- 1 cup of hummus
- 2 bell peppers, sliced into strips
- 2 carrots, sliced into sticks
- 2 celery stalks, sliced into sticks
- 1 cup cherry tomatoes
- 1 cup cucumber slices
- Handful of snap peas
- Salt and pepper to taste
- 1 tablespoon olive oil

Instructions:

1. Wash all vegetables and pat them dry with a paper towel.

2. Prepare the hummus by blending 1 cup of chickpeas, 2 cloves of garlic, 2 tablespoons of tahini, 1 tablespoon of lemon juice, and 1 tablespoon of olive oil in a food processor until smooth. Add a little bit of water if the consistency is too thick.

3. Season the hummus with salt and pepper to taste.

4. In a frying pan, heat 1 tablespoon of olive oil over medium-high heat.

5. Add the sliced bell peppers and cook for 2-3 minutes until they become slightly soft.

6. Add the sliced carrots and celery and cook for another 2 minutes.

7. Once the vegetables are slightly soft, remove them from heat and let them cool.

8. Arrange the cooked vegetable strips, cherry tomatoes, cucumber slices, and snap peas on a serving platter.

9. Place the hummus in a small bowl in the center of the platter.

10. Serve the platter with whole wheat pita bread or your choice of whole grain crackers.

11. Enjoy your healthy and delicious Veggie and Hummus Platter! Remember to adjust the portion sizes of each vegetable according to your individual dietary needs. This platter is high in fiber and low in carbohydrates, making it a great option for type 2 diabetes patients. It's also packed with essential vitamins and nutrients from the colorful array of vegetables.

Related Book [Type 1 Diabetes Cookbook For Kids, Teens, Women, Men And Adults](#) **By Caroline Johnson**

Baked Sweet Potato Chips

Ingredients:
- 2 medium-sized sweet potatoes
- 1 tablespoon of olive oil
- 1 teaspoon of salt
- 1 teaspoon of garlic powder
- 1 teaspoon of onion powder
- 1 teaspoon of paprika
- 1/4 teaspoon of black pepper

Instructions:

1. Preheat your oven to 375 degrees Fahrenheit (190 degrees Celsius).

2. Peel the sweet potatoes and slice them as thinly as possible, about 1/8 inch thick. You can use a sharp knife or a mandolin slicer for even slices.

3. In a small bowl, mix together all the seasonings: salt, garlic powder, onion powder, paprika, and black pepper. Set aside.

4. In a large mixing bowl, add the sliced sweet potatoes and drizzle with olive oil. Toss gently to make sure the sweet potato slices are evenly coated with oil.

5. Sprinkle the seasoning mixture over the sweet potatoes and toss again to ensure each slice is coated with the seasonings.

6. Line a baking sheet with parchment paper and arrange the seasoned sweet potato slices in a single layer on the sheet.

7. Bake in the preheated oven for 15-20 minutes, flipping halfway through, until the sweet potato chips are crispy and lightly browned.

8. Let the chips cool for a few minutes before serving. Enjoy as a healthy snack option for type 2 diabetes patients.

Tips:

- You can adjust the seasonings to your preference. For a spicier version, add cayenne pepper or chili powder.
- Make sure to slice the sweet potatoes as thinly as possible for a crispy texture.
- Store any leftover chips in an airtight container for up to 2 days. Reheat in the oven at 375 degrees Fahrenheit (190 degrees Celsius) for 5-10 minutes before serving.

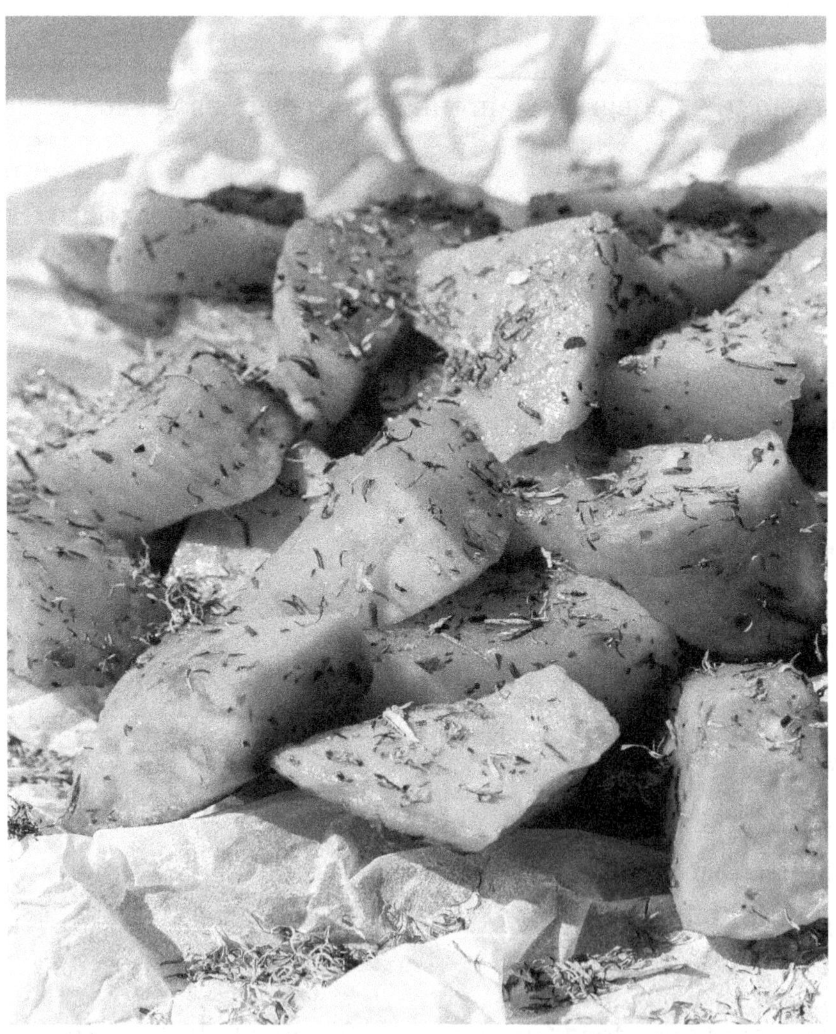

Chocolate Avocado Pudding

Ingredients:

- 1 ripe avocado
- ¼ cup unsweetened cocoa powder
- 2 tablespoons of sugar-free sweetener
- ½ cup unsweetened almond milk
- 1 teaspoon vanilla extract
- 1 tablespoon of unsalted almond butter
- Optional toppings: sliced almonds, dark chocolate chips

Instructions:

1. Cut the avocado in half, remove the seed, and scoop the flesh out into a blender or food processor.

2. Add the cocoa powder, sugar-free sweetener, almond milk, vanilla extract, and almond butter to the blender/food processor with the avocado.

3. Blend all the ingredients until the mixture is smooth and creamy.

4. If the pudding is too thick, add a splash of almond milk to thin it out.

5. Transfer the chocolate avocado pudding to a bowl or individual serving cups.

6. If desired, sprinkle sliced almonds and/or dark chocolate chips on top of the pudding for added flavor and crunch.

7. Refrigerate for at least 30 minutes to allow the pudding to thicken and chill.

8. Serve and enjoy your delicious and nutritious chocolate avocado pudding!

Nutritional information (per serving):

Calories: 196

Carbohydrates: 14g

Protein: 4g

Fat: 16g

Fiber: 7g

Sugars: 3g

Note: This recipe can be modified to suit personal preferences and dietary restrictions. If you are lactose intolerant, you can substitute the almond milk with a dairy-free alternative like coconut milk. You can also add in other toppings like fresh berries or a dollop of sugar-free whipped cream. Remember to always consult with a doctor or registered dietitian before making significant changes to your diet plan. Enjoy in moderation as part of a well-balanced diet.

Berry and Yogurt Parfait

Ingredients:

- 1 cup plain Greek yogurt

- 1 cup fresh berries (such as strawberries, blueberries, raspberries)

- 1/4 cup chopped nuts (such as almonds, walnuts, or pecans)

- 1/4 cup sugar-free granola

- 1 tsp honey (optional)

- 1 tsp cinnamon (optional)

Instructions:

1. Prepare the berries: Wash the fresh berries and pat them dry. Slice the strawberries into small pieces and keep the blueberries and raspberries whole.

2. Assemble the parfait: Begin by layering half of the Greek yogurt in a glass or mason jar. Next, add half of the sliced strawberries and blueberries on top of the yogurt. Then sprinkle half of the chopped nuts and sugar-free granola on the berries.

3. Repeat the layering: Add another layer of Greek yogurt on top of the nuts and granola. Then layer the remaining berries on top of the yogurt. Finally, sprinkle the rest of the nuts and granola on the berries.

4. Optional: For added sweetness and flavor, you can drizzle a teaspoon of honey on top of the parfait and sprinkle some cinnamon.

5. Serve and enjoy: Your berry and yogurt parfait is now ready to be enjoyed! This parfait can also be prepared ahead of time and stored in the fridge for a healthy and convenient breakfast or snack option.

Nutrition information (per serving):

Calories: 250

Carbohydrates: 20g

Protein: 14g

Fat: 12g

Fiber: 5g

Sodium: 50mg

Note: This recipe is suitable for individuals with type 2 diabetes as it contains healthy and balanced ingredients with low sugar and carbohydrates. It can also be modified by using low-fat yogurt or skipping the honey to reduce the calories and carbohydrates even further.

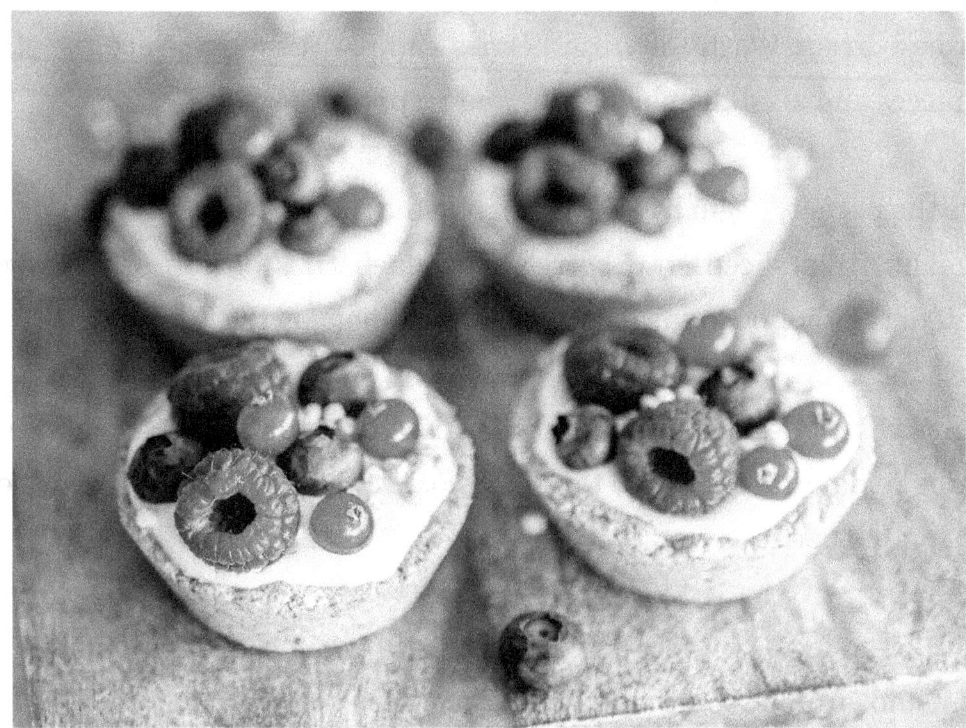

Baked Apples with Cinnamon and Pecans

Ingredients:

- 4 apples (Honeycrisp or Granny Smith work best)

- 1 tsp ground cinnamon

- 1/4 cup chopped pecans

- 2 tbsp coconut oil or butter, melted

- 2 tbsp sugar-free maple syrup (or regular maple syrup if desired)

- 1/4 cup water

- Optional: sugar-free vanilla ice cream or whipped cream for serving

Instructions:

1. Preheat your oven to 375°F (190°C).

2. Rinse and dry the apples. Cut off the top of the apples (about ½ inch) and remove the core, leaving the bottom intact. Use a spoon or melon baller to hollow out the apples, leaving about ½ inch of the flesh intact.

3. In a small bowl, mix together the melted coconut oil (or butter), sugar-free maple syrup, and ground cinnamon.

4. In a separate bowl, mix together the chopped pecans and 2 tablespoons of the coconut oil/maple syrup mixture.

5. Place the hollowed-out apples in a baking dish and pour the remaining coconut oil/maple syrup mixture into the middle of each apple.

6. Stuff the chopped pecan mixture into the center of each apple.

7. Pour ¼ cup of water into the bottom of the baking dish. This will help the apples stay moist while baking.

8. Bake the apples for 30-35 minutes, or until they are soft and the filling is golden brown.

9. Optional: Serve the baked apples with a scoop of sugar-free vanilla ice cream or a dollop of whipped cream on top.

10. Enjoy your delicious and healthy Baked Apples with Cinnamon and Pecans! Because it is a dessert with natural sweetness and high in fiber, it can be a great treat for type 2 diabetes patients. Just make sure to monitor your blood sugar levels and adjust the portion size accordingly.

Visit Caroline Johnson Author Central page for more health books

Banana and Peanut Butter "Ice Cream"

Ingredients:
- 2 ripe bananas
- 2 tablespoons of all-natural peanut butter
- 1 teaspoon of vanilla extract
- 1/4 teaspoon of cinnamon
- 1/8 teaspoon of salt (optional)

Instructions:

1. Peel the bananas and cut them into small chunks. Place them in a single layer on a baking sheet lined with parchment paper.
2. Freeze the banana chunks for at least 2 hours or overnight.
3. Once frozen, add the bananas, peanut butter, vanilla extract, cinnamon, and salt (if using) into a blender or food processor.
4. Blend the mixture until it becomes smooth and creamy. If the consistency is too thick, you can add 1-2 tablespoons of almond milk to help loosen it up.
5. Transfer the mixture into a container and freeze it for at least 1 hour to let it firm up.
6. Serve the banana and peanut butter "ice cream" in a bowl or cone and enjoy!
7. You can also top it with some chopped nuts or dark chocolate chips for an extra crunch.

Nutrition Facts (per serving):
- Calories: 170
- Carbohydrates: 22g
- Fat: 9g
- Protein: 4g
- Fiber: 3g
- Sugar: 10g

Tips:

- You can use different varieties of nut butter such as almond butter or cashew butter to switch up the flavor.
- You can also add in some dark chocolate chips or unsweetened cocoa powder to make it a chocolate peanut butter "ice cream."
- For a vegan option, use almond or coconut milk instead of dairy milk.
- This recipe can also be used as a topping for waffles, pancakes, or oatmeal for a delicious and healthy breakfast option.

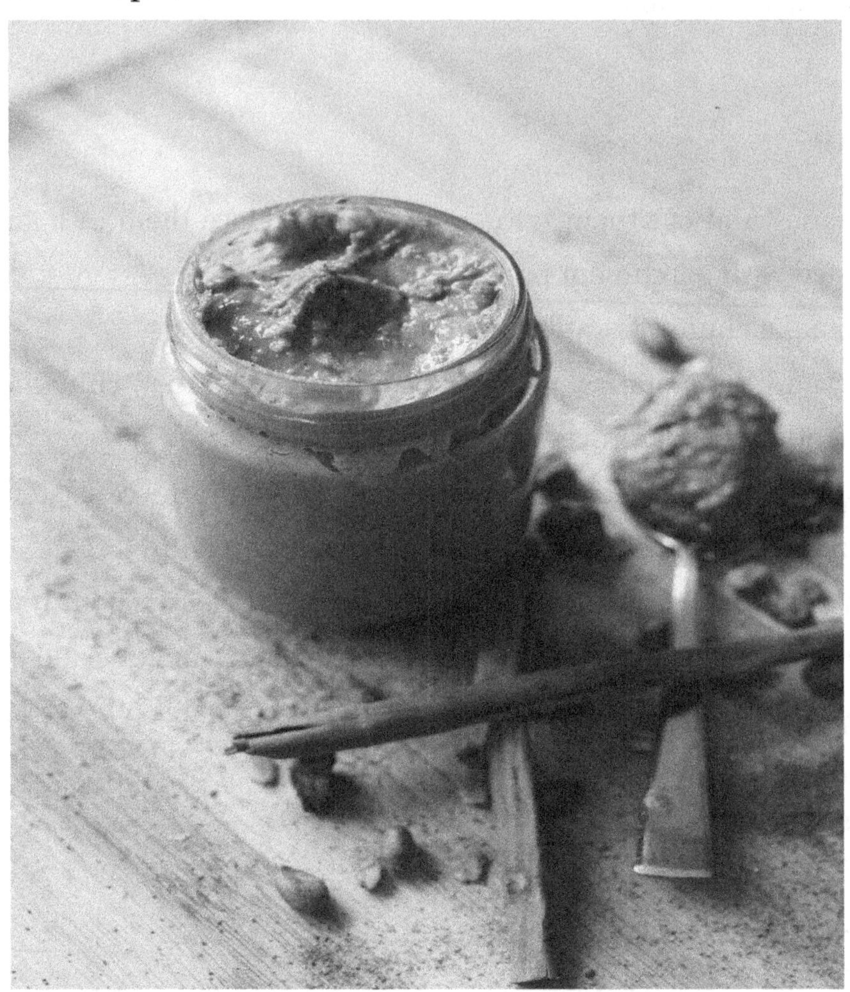

Part 8: Meal Planning and Preparation Tips

Weekly Meal Plan

Week 1

Monday:

Breakfast: Egg and vegetable scramble with whole wheat toast

Snack: Greek yogurt with berries

Lunch: Grilled chicken salad with avocado, tomatoes, and balsamic dressing

Snack: Apple slices with natural peanut butter

Dinner: Baked fish with roasted vegetables and quinoa

Tuesday:

Breakfast: Overnight oats with almond milk, chia seeds, and topped with almonds and cinnamon

Snack: Carrots and cucumber slices with hummus

Lunch: Turkey and cheese wrap with whole wheat tortilla, cucumber, and avocado

Snack: Hard-boiled egg and a small apple

Dinner: Lean beef stir-fry with brown rice and steamed broccoli

Wednesday:

Breakfast: Whole grain English muffin with scrambled eggs and spinach

Snack: Sugar-free Greek yogurt with a handful of almonds

Lunch: Lentil soup with a side of mixed greens salad with olive oil and lemon dressing

Snack: Celery sticks with natural peanut butter

Dinner: Grilled tofu with roasted sweet potatoes and green beans

Thursday:

Breakfast: Spinach and mushroom omelette with whole wheat toast

Snack: Low-fat cheese stick and a small orange

Lunch: Quinoa and black bean salad with mixed vegetables

Snack: Handful of baby carrots and sugar-free ranch dip

Dinner: Baked chicken breast with steamed asparagus and a side of whole grain pasta with marinara sauce

Friday:
Breakfast: Whole wheat waffles topped with berries and a side of turkey bacon
Snack: Small bowl of fresh fruit salad
Lunch: Grilled salmon with roasted Brussels sprouts and a side of brown rice
Snack: Hard-boiled egg and a small handful of almonds
Dinner: Vegetable stir-fry with tofu and brown rice

Saturday:
Breakfast: Whole grain toast with avocado and a poached egg on top
Snack: Sugar-free yogurt with mixed berries
Lunch: Grilled shrimp and vegetable skewers with quinoa
Snack: Small apple with natural peanut butter
Dinner: Baked fish with a side of roasted root vegetables and a small green salad with oil and vinegar dressing

Sunday:
Breakfast: Vegetable and cheese omelette with a side of whole wheat toast
Snack: Hummus and vegetable platter
Lunch: Grilled chicken breast with a mixed greens salad and balsamic dressing
Snack: Air-popped popcorn
Dinner: Quinoa-stuffed peppers with lean ground turkey and steamed broccoli on the side.

Week 2
Monday:
Breakfast: Greek yogurt with fresh berries and a sprinkle of flaxseeds
Lunch: Grilled chicken salad with mixed greens, cucumbers, tomatoes, and avocado
Dinner: Baked salmon with steamed broccoli and quinoa

Tuesday:

Breakfast: Oatmeal with almond milk, chopped apples, and a sprinkle of cinnamon

Lunch: Turkey and vegetable wrap with whole wheat tortilla and hummus

Dinner: Vegetarian chili with black beans, tomatoes, kale, and bell peppers

Wednesday:

Breakfast: Spinach and mushroom omelette with whole grain toast

Lunch: Tuna salad with whole wheat crackers and cucumber slices

Dinner: Grilled shrimp skewers with zucchini and bell peppers, served with brown rice

Thursday:

Breakfast: Whole grain toast with avocado and boiled eggs

Lunch: Quinoa and black bean bowl with roasted sweet potatoes and corn

Dinner: Baked chicken breast with roasted Brussels sprouts and cauliflower mash

Friday:

Breakfast: Smoothie made with almond milk, spinach, banana, and chia seeds

Lunch: Veggie and hummus wrap with a side of carrot and celery sticks

Dinner: Baked tofu with roasted asparagus and a mixed grain pilaf

Saturday:

Breakfast: Whole grain pancakes with fresh fruit and sugar-free syrup

Lunch: Grilled vegetable and feta quinoa salad

Dinner: Baked fish with roasted vegetables and a side of whole grain pasta with marinara sauce

Sunday:

Breakfast: Poached eggs with whole grain toast and steamed spinach

Lunch: Lentil soup with a side of whole grain crackers and a side salad

Dinner: Grilled lean steak with roasted sweet potatoes and steamed green beans.

Week 3

Monday:

Breakfast:

- Oatmeal with almond milk, topped with berries and a sprinkle of cinnamon

- Whole grain toast with avocado and boiled egg

- Unsweetened green tea

Lunch:

- Grilled chicken breast salad with mixed greens, cherry tomatoes, cucumbers, and a homemade vinaigrette dressing

- Small whole grain pita bread

- Greek yogurt with a handful of mixed nuts

Dinner:

- Baked salmon with lemon and herbs, served with roasted vegetables and quinoa

- Small side salad with balsamic vinaigrette dressing

- Sparkling water with a splash of lemon

Snack:

- Celery sticks with hummus

- Small handful of unsalted almonds

Tuesday:

Breakfast:

- Scrambled eggs with spinach and feta cheese

- Whole grain English muffin with a thin spread of butter or avocado

- Fresh squeezed orange juice

Lunch:

- Turkey and cheese whole wheat wrap with lettuce, tomatoes, and cucumber

- Small apple

- Sparkling water with a splash of orange juice

Dinner:

- Grilled chicken kebabs with bell peppers, onions, and mushrooms
- Small side of brown rice
- Steamed broccoli
- Low-fat Greek yogurt with fresh fruit for dessert

Snack:

- Small whole grain crackers with cheese slices
- Carrot sticks with hummus

Wednesday:
Breakfast:

- Vegetable and cheese omelet
- Whole grain toast with a thin spread of peanut butter
- Unsweetened herbal tea

Lunch:

- Quinoa and black bean salad with diced tomatoes, corn, and avocado
- Small whole grain pita bread
- Sparkling water with a splash of lime juice

Dinner:

- Grilled pork chop with roasted sweet potatoes and Brussels sprouts
- Small side salad with balsamic vinaigrette dressing
- Fresh berries with a dollop of whipped cream for dessert

Snack:

- Air-popped popcorn
- Small bowl of mixed fruit

Thursday:
Breakfast:

- Greek yogurt with fresh berries and a sprinkle of granola

- Hard-boiled egg

- Unsweetened green tea

Lunch:

- Tuna salad sandwich with whole grain bread, lettuce, and tomato

- Small side of carrot sticks and bell pepper slices

- Sparkling water with a splash of lemon

Dinner:

- Grilled shrimp with zucchini noodles and marinara sauce

- Small side of whole grain garlic bread

- Steamed asparagus

- Low-fat ice cream for dessert

Snack:

- Small apple with almond butter

- Small handful of trail mix

Friday:

Breakfast:

- Avocado toast with an egg on top

- Fresh fruit salad

- Unsweetened herbal tea

Lunch:

- Grilled chicken Caesar salad with whole wheat croutons

- Clementine

- Sparkling water with a splash of cranberry juice

Dinner:

- Baked fish with a lemon butter sauce, served with roasted vegetables and a small side of whole grain pasta
- Small side salad with balsamic vinaigrette dressing
- Small piece of dark chocolate for dessert

Snack:
- Small whole grain crackers with tuna salad
- Small bowl of grapes

Saturday:
Breakfast:
- Whole grain pancakes with sugar-free syrup and fresh fruit
- Turkey bacon
- Unsweetened green tea

Lunch:
- Black bean and veggie burger on a whole wheat bun, served with a side of sweet potato fries
- Small side salad with balsamic vinaigrette dressing
- Sparkling water with a splash of orange juice

Dinner:
- Grilled chicken breast with sautéed spinach and quinoa pilaf
- Small side of steamed carrots
- Low-fat frozen yogurt for dessert

Snack:
- Small pear with cheese slices
- Small handful of walnuts

Sunday:
Breakfast:

- Egg white veggie omelette
- Whole grain toast with a thin spread of butter or avocado
- Fresh squeezed orange juice

Lunch:
- Grilled vegetable and hummus wrap
- Small side of fresh fruit
- Sparkling water with a splash of lime juice

Dinner:
- Baked turkey meatballs with whole wheat spaghetti and tomato sauce
- Small side salad with balsamic vinaigrette dressing
- Steamed green beans
- Fresh berries with a dollop of whipped cream for dessert

Snack:
- Small whole grain crackers with cheese slices
- Small apple with peanut butter dip

Remember to always consult with a doctor or registered dietitian for personalized meal plans and guidance for managing type 2 diabetes.

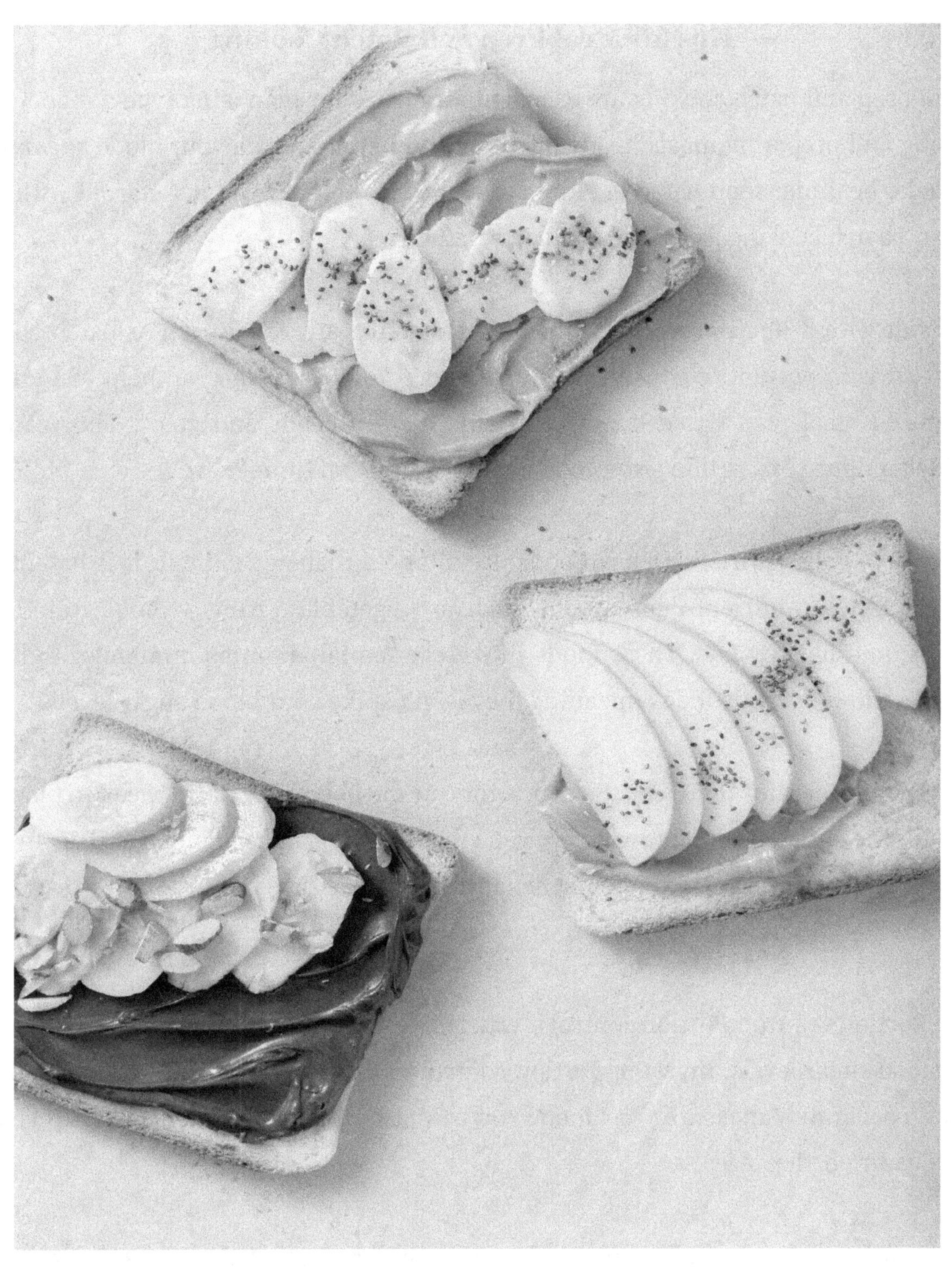

Tips for Meal Prep and Batch Cooking

Meal prep and batch cooking are excellent strategies for managing type 2 diabetes. By planning and preparing meals in advance, you can better control your blood sugar levels and make healthier food choices. Here are some tips to help you get started with meal prep and batch cooking as a type 2 diabetes patient:

1. Consult with a Registered Dietitian: Before starting any meal prep or batch cooking routine, it is important to consult with a registered dietitian who can help you create a customized meal plan based on your specific dietary needs and goals. They can also provide guidance on portion sizes, food choices, and meal timing.

2. Choose Whole, Nutrient-Dense Foods: As a type 2 diabetes patient, it is essential to focus on whole, nutrient-dense foods such as vegetables, fruits, whole grains, lean proteins, and healthy fats. These foods provide essential vitamins, minerals, and fiber, and have a low glycemic index, meaning they won't spike your blood sugar levels.

3. Plan Your Meals for the Week: Set aside time at the beginning of the week to plan your meals for the entire week. This will help you create a well-balanced menu and ensure that you have all the necessary ingredients on hand. It will also save you time and stress during the week.

4. Use Portion Control: Portion control is crucial for managing diabetes, as it helps control your blood sugar levels. Invest in portion control tools such as measuring cups and food scales to accurately measure your food. You can also use smaller plates to help visually control your portion sizes.

5. Cook in Bulk: Batch cooking involves preparing large quantities of food at once and storing it in the refrigerator or freezer for future meals. This is a great way to save time and effort, and it ensures that you always have healthy meals on hand. Make sure to properly label and store your cooked meals to avoid confusion and food waste.

6. Incorporate Variety and Balance: Eating a variety of foods is not only important for your physical health but also for your mental well-being. Try to incorporate a variety of flavors, textures, and colors into your meals to keep things interesting and enjoyable. Also, make sure to include a balance of carbohydrates, proteins, and healthy fats in each meal.

7. Opt for Healthy Cooking Methods: How you cook your food can significantly impact its nutritional value. Avoid deep-frying or using excess oil, and opt for healthier cooking methods such as grilling, baking, steaming, or broiling. These methods help retain the nutrients in your food without adding excess unhealthy fats.

8. Don't Forget Snacks: It is important to have healthy snacks on hand to prevent blood sugar dips between meals. Include snacks like fresh fruits, nuts, and protein-rich foods like hard-boiled eggs or hummus and vegetables. Prep these in advance and portion them out to make snacking convenient and healthy.

9. Invest in Meal Prep Containers: Having the right containers is key for meal prep and batch cooking. Invest in BPA-free, leak-proof, and microwave-safe containers to store your meals. This will help keep your food fresh, make heating up meals easier, and prevent any mess.

10. Involve Your Family: Meal prep and batch cooking can be a fun and educational experience for the whole family. Involve your family members in planning and cooking meals. This will not only help you save time and energy, but it can also encourage healthier eating habits for the whole family.

By following these tips, you can make meal prep and batch cooking a successful and sustainable part of your diabetes management plan. Remember to always listen to your body, monitor your blood sugar levels, and make adjustments as needed. With a little planning and preparation, you can take charge of your diabetes and make healthy eating simple and enjoyable.

Conclusion

In conclusion, the journey towards managing and controlling type 2 diabetes may seem daunting, but with the right tools and resources, it is possible to live a healthy and fulfilling life. The "Type 2 Diabetes Cookbook for Beginners" is a comprehensive guide that aims to equip individuals with the knowledge and skills to make better food choices and manage their condition effectively.

The cookbook provides a plethora of recipes, meal plans, and essential information about type 2 diabetes. It emphasizes the importance of a well-balanced diet, consisting of whole, unprocessed foods, and the avoidance of sugary and refined products. It also encourages regular physical activity, which plays a crucial role in maintaining blood sugar levels and overall health.

One of the key takeaways from this cookbook is the emphasis on incorporating fresh, nutrient-dense ingredients into your meals. This not only provides essential vitamins and minerals but also helps in managing weight, a vital factor in type 2 diabetes management. The book also features quick and easy recipes, perfect for individuals with busy lifestyles, ensuring that healthy eating becomes a sustainable part of their routine.

Moreover, the "Type 2 Diabetes Cookbook for Beginners" offers valuable tips and advice on how to navigate social gatherings and dining out while managing the condition. This is.

Apart from providing delicious and nutritious recipes, the cookbook also emphasizes the importance of self-care and self-monitoring. This includes regularly checking blood sugar levels and keeping track of food intake. It also encourages readers to seek support from family, friends, and healthcare professionals, addressing the emotional and mental aspect of living with type 2 diabetes.

Visit Caroline Johnson Author Central page for more health books